The
Diabetes Diet

DR. BERNSTEIN'S
LOW-CARBOHYDRATE SOLUTION

Also by Richard K. Bernstein, M.D.

Dr. Bernstein's Diabetes Solution

*Diabetes: The Glucograf Method
for Normalizing Blood Sugar*

Diabetes Type II

The
Diabetes Diet

DR. BERNSTEIN'S
LOW-CARBOHYDRATE SOLUTION

**Richard K. Bernstein, M.D.,
F.A.C.E., F.A.C.N., C.W.S.**

Recipes by Marcia Miele

LITTLE, BROWN AND COMPANY

NEW YORK   BOSTON   LONDON

Little, Brown and Company
Hachette Book Group USA
237 Park Avenue, New York, NY 10017

Visit our Web site at www.HachetteBookGroupUSA.com

First Edition: January 2005

AUTHOR'S NOTE
This book is not intended as a substitute for professional medical care. The reader should regularly consult a physician for all health-related problems and routine care.

Library of Congress Cataloging-in-Publication Data

Bernstein, Richard K.
  The diabetes diet : Dr. Bernstein's low-carbohydrate solution / Richard K. Bernstein.
      p. cm.
  Includes index.
  ISBN 978-0-316-73784-5
  1. Diabetes — Diet therapy — Recipes.   2. Low-carbohydrate diet — Recipes.   I. Title.

RC662.B417   2005
616.4'620654 — dc22   2004011739

10 9 8 7 6 5 4 3

Q-FF

Printed in the United States of America

Contents

v

Contents

Author's Note

It is no exaggeration to say that the Diabetes Diet is a life-saver. Indeed, I believe I can make a claim that no other diet author can — that my own diet saved my life. I'm not the only one. Patients have raved about the new health and vigor they've found by using my diet. There's a reason why diabetics, the overweight, and the obese have suddenly got control of their lives with this plan: it works.

Six months ago I went to my fiftieth college class reunion. I was one of two people present who were still recognizable from half a century before. The other one plays tennis a couple hours every day. I was the only person in my original class with type 1 diabetes. Unlike most everyone there, I was considerably healthier fifty years after college than during it.

Many of my former classmates sported coronary bypass scars — I'd guess that out of 150 people there, about a third had undergone bypass surgery. Others were obese. Most appeared much older than I. Why them and not me? In college I would never have thought this would be the case. By the time I graduated, I'd been a type 1 diabetic for almost half my life. I already had many complications of the disease. Eventually, seeking to arrest the downward spiral of my health, I came to analyze virtually everything I ate, constantly monitoring the effects on my blood sugars and my health. This is also a claim most diet doctors probably cannot make, and it provides me with an utterly distinct view of how diet affects not only me, but people in general. I would not necessarily wish my particular vantage point on anyone, but it has given me insights that I never would have had otherwise. The key insight was that what I ate as a young man nearly killed me.

I would surmise that my classmates had mostly not aged well because they had stuck to the conventional wisdom on diet. Who could blame them? If you can't trust your doctor, whom can you trust?

Yet I can safely say that I am healthier today because I did *not* trust my doctor, who had told me that what I have accomplished would not be possible. I can also say that I am healthier today not *in spite* of having a potentially fatal illness, but *because* of it.

Although I'm now in my seventies, many doctors would mistake my health profile for that of a much younger man. When I was on a very low fat, high-carbohydrate diet more than thirty years ago, I had high fasting triglycerides (usually over 250 mg/dl) and high serum cholesterol (usually over 300 mg/dl), and I developed a number of vascular and other complications. When I went onto a very low carbohydrate diet and did not restrict my fat, my lipids plummeted (lipids are fatty substances in the blood). It's not an exaggeration to say that through this low-carbohydrate diet plan, I achieved the lipid profile of an Olympic athlete, merely as the result of trying to normalize my blood sugars. That I exercised regularly certainly didn't hurt my lipid profile — but I was also exercising when my lipid profile was abnormal.

Dare your physician. Ask if the lipid profile of anyone he or she knows on a low-fat diet can remotely compare to what I had achieved on a low-carbohydrate diet with unrestricted fats:

- LDL — the "bad" cholesterol — 63 (below 100 is considered normal)
- HDL — the "good" cholesterol — 116 (above 40 is considered normal)
- Triglycerides — 45 (below 150 is considered normal)
- Lipoprotein(a) — undetectable (below 30 is considered normal)

Contrary to popular myth, fat is not a demon. It's the body's way of storing energy and maintaining essential organs such as the brain. Without essential fatty acids your body would cease to function.

It's an odd twist of fate that I am likely much healthier now than I would have been had I not been a diabetic. The diet is why.

The diet presented in these pages was originally designed as a diabetes diet — and as effective as it has been for countless diabetics, it is much more than just that. Indeed, as more information has become available over the last two decades on the toxic nature of a high-carbohydrate diet, it has never been clearer that the benefits of this diet are nearly as profound for those who do not have diabetes as for those who do.

We see the consequences of the standard American diet, or SAD, all around us: the dramatic public health burden of a society two-thirds of whose members are overweight.

Health care costs are soaring, and they will continue to do so, with as many as 20 million Americans suffering from diagnosed and undiagnosed diabetes. There is a desperate race for a cure, when in fact the largest percentage of diabetics could have the same kind of excellent health I have enjoyed if they followed this diet's prescription.

In my practice I see the very personal consequences of SAD: from the social stigma of obesity to life-threatening issues of heart disease and stroke to sexual dysfunction — the list goes on.

Regardless of whether you are slim or obese, fit or fat, old or young, this diet will promote health and longevity. I recommend following it your whole life, as I now do, in order to enjoy the kinds of benefits I have seen. Even over the short term it can benefit your life and health. Studies have shown that normalizing blood sugars for periods as brief as two weeks can have lasting benefits. So there is every reason to believe that even if you don't feel that you can stick to it forever — which is, of course, what I recommend — sticking to it for as long as possible can have significant benefits. My belief, however, is that you will be so pleased with the results you won't want to go back to SAD.

I invite you to be well. I invite you to live long, eat well, and enjoy a healthy, vigorous life.

Acknowledgments

I would like to express my sincere appreciation to Stephen Stark, novelist, editor, and friend, for his insight and encouragement. Steve's many suggestions, not only about the narrative of this book but also about the recipes (he knows his way around a kitchen much better than I), were invaluable.

I am grateful to my editor, Elizabeth Nagle, for adding a professional touch to the narrative without imposing any significant deletions and especially for her efforts to upgrade the cover art. Patricia A. Gian and Anne E. Bernstein, M.D., reviewed the manuscript and suggested many improvements. Channa Taub, literary agent nonpareil, initially conceived the idea for this book and coaxed me into undertaking this endeavor despite my time commitment to the clinical treatment of diabetes.

Executive copyeditor Peggy Leith Anderson was the last person to cope with the manuscript, and as for my last two books, she did a superb job, facilitating my final review and saving me the embarrassment of many ambiguities and even mistakes.

The

Diabetes Diet

Dr. Bernstein's
Low-Carbohydrate Solution

Introduction

Whenever I see a celebrity battling obesity — yo-yo dieting or having dangerous gastric bypass surgery — I think, *It doesn't have to be.*

In my experience nearly every obese person I've treated, whether clinically diagnosed with diabetes or not, has elevated blood sugars and will face the complications of diabetes.

Whenever I hear the news that a celebrity — or anyone else for that matter — has died as the result of the complications of diabetes, my first thought is: *It didn't have to happen.*

Johnny Cash, Jackie Robinson, Nikita Khrushchev, and Ella Fitzgerald died from complications of diabetes. Aretha Franklin and Mary Tyler Moore are diabetics. Ray Kroc, the man you could safely call the godfather of fast food — and who may have indirectly contributed to the diabetes of millions of Americans — was himself a diabetic. Tragically, his daughter also had diabetes, and died much younger than he did. Chances are good that if she could have known back then, in the late 1960s and early 1970s,

3

what I know now, she might still be alive — and not only alive but healthy.

I know, because the statistics said that I should have been dead by 1976.

When I was diagnosed with type 1 diabetes in 1946, the life expectancy after diagnosis of diabetics like me was about thirty years. My death would not have come from diabetes per se. I am pretty certain that I would have died of kidney failure, a direct result of the low-fat, high-carbohydrate, American Diabetes Association (ADA) diet I followed for twenty-four years after my diagnosis.

In the late 1960s I discovered considerable protein in my urine. At that time there was no kidney dialysis and there were no kidney transplants. I read that this amount of protein in my urine meant one thing: advanced kidney disease. Kidneys filter the blood of toxic substances, and protein in my urine meant that soon enough my body would drown itself in poison. Back in engineering school, a classmate had told me how his nondiabetic sister had died of kidney disease. Before her death she had ballooned with retained water, and I began to have nightmares of blowing up like a balloon.

I had been twelve years old in 1946, when I was diagnosed with diabetes. By the late 1960s to mid-1970s, I was married and had small children. Although I was in what is for most people the prime of life, my body was like an old man's. I'd had excruciatingly painful kidney stones, a stone in a salivary duct, stones in my gallbladder, and "frozen" shoulders. Not only had my feet become progressively deformed, they had begun to lose sensation from peripheral neuropathy, the kind of nerve damage that could eventually lead to amputation. After a routine exercise stress test, I was told that my heart had been damaged — scar tissue had replaced muscle tissue (a condition known as cardiomyopathy), a common cause of heart failure and death among type 1 diabetics.

When I would mention these problems to my diabetologist, who was then president of the ADA, he usually told me, "Don't worry, it has nothing to do with your diabetes. You're doing fine." I wasn't doing fine, of course. Still, in one sense my doctor was right. My diabetes didn't have to lead to such complications. The right diet could have controlled my blood sugars, but he didn't know that. At that time I didn't know it either. At that time the life expectancy of a person with advanced kidney disease was around five years. I was deeply frustrated that I could not solve the problem of my own disease. There is a saying among engineers that there is no such thing as a problem without a solution. Engineers also know that you need tools to solve problems, and if you don't have them you often have to invent them — or find new uses for tools that already exist.

As an engineer I was accustomed to being presented with difficult problems, which, if attacked piece by piece, could be solved. I was the one, however, who was being attacked piece by piece.

I WILL GLADLY ADMIT that back in 1969, I was as affected by the conventional thinking as anyone and had no idea that the result I was looking for was normalized blood sugars.

I was lucky. Right around the time I was certain my life was near its end, I got a second chance and was fortunate enough to make the most of it.

That year I happened across an ad in a scientific journal for the first blood sugar meter. Although virtually every diabetic has at least one nowadays, back then they were brand-new. Indeed, its manufacturer had intended it as a piece of machinery to be sold to doctors and hospitals, a niche product that could read blood sugar levels in 1 minute from a single drop of blood. In that capacity, it was a potential lifesaver. People who lose consciousness due to very high blood sugar (ketoacidosis) from diabetes give off an odor that can be mistaken for the odor of alcohol. Before the blood sugar meter was developed, many unconscious diabetics died if they happened to end up in the emergency room after laboratory hours. Mistaken for drunks, some were allowed to sleep it off, right into eternity.

I wish I could say that as soon as I saw the blood sugar meter I had an epiphany and knew at once that the device could turn my life around, along with the lives of millions of other diabetics. It was more like coming across the Ark of the Covenant and thinking it looked pretty comfortable. Which is to say that while I knew it was going to be useful, I had no idea how important it would really be.

I'd had my share of low blood sugar episodes, a condition called hypoglycemia, which can begin with irritability and end in unconsciousness. My family didn't find me terribly charming when I was irritable, and was terrified when I was unconscious. I had the idea that if I got one of these machines, I could measure my blood sugars and, if they got low, bring them up.

I tried to get a blood sugar meter, but the manufacturer would sell them only to doctors or hospitals. If my wife had not been a physician, I might have gone on and died, but she was, and I obtained one through her. It cost $650, in those days a hefty sum. At the very least, you could have bought a pretty good used car.

In short order I became the first diabetic patient to

monitor his own blood sugar levels. While I used the machine for my original intent, to catch hypoglycemic episodes early, I also began to discover the effects that various foods had on my blood sugar. Engineers solve problems mathematically, but you have to know the mechanics of a problem in order to solve it. Now, for the first time, I was gaining insight into the mechanics and mathematics of my disease. What I learned in my frequent testing was that my own blood sugars swung from very low to very high about twice daily. The blood sugar meter quickly became an indispensable tool.

The hormone insulin has two main effects, as we'll discuss in more detail further on. first, it's the key that unlocks our body's cells to allow glucose in, second, it's the major fat-building hormone. I (like other type 1 diabetics) was skinny because of chronically high blood sugars that I could not adequately control with injected insulin. I could not get glucose into my cells in order to use it.

Three years of blood sugar testing went by, and although I was aware of my blood sugars levels daily, I was still the proverbial "98-pound weakling," wracked with complications. I was eating the same food and taking the same medication for my symptoms — still not connecting the dots between the foods that I ate and my blood sugar roller coaster.

I was more than frustrated. First and foremost was the life and death issue — by the measure of kidney disease, I had only a few years left — but there was also an intellectual issue. I knew there was something more. I suspected that the answer to reversing diabetic complications would be exercise.

I ordered a search of the medical literature on diabetic complications and exercise. In the early 1970s this was not a matter of searching keywords on Google. It was more like going to the library and looking up a subject in the catalog of periodicals, then examining the results on microfilm. Except the information I was looking for wasn't so readily available. I had to send away for a search of the literature.

What I found when I got the results of my $75 search was that my hypothesis was wrong. There was nothing on exercise helping with diabetic complications. So — as an engineer — I had left my hypothesis in serious doubt. But I discovered what the answer was. The results of my search, which took weeks to arrive, were several studies on *blood sugar normalization* in animals, and how *it,* not exercise, helped reverse diabetic complications. If I had a eureka moment, this was it.

When I showed these results to my doctor, he was not impressed. If he was even intrigued, he did not show it. "Animals are different," was his response. Anyway, blood sugar normalization, he told me, was impossible in humans.

So I took up my quest alone. I spent the next year checking my blood sugars 5–8 times each day. Every few days I'd make a small, experimental change in my diet or insulin regimen to see what the effect would be on my blood sugar. If a change brought an improvement, I'd retain it. If it made blood sugars worse, I'd discard it. Invariably I found that the foods I had been told to emphasize — carbohydrates — were those that caused rapid and substantial rises in blood sugar. Those I had been told to avoid — protein and fats — were the ones that had a much less profound and rapid effect.

On a graph my blood sugar swings on the high-carbohydrate diet would look like sharp peaks and valleys. I discovered that with a low-carbohydrate diet, they were much closer to a somewhat wavy line. I also discovered that what had been true in the animal studies was true for me: my complications began to ease. Despite the disdain of my doctor for my tinkering, the protein disappeared from my urine. Other complications gradually evaporated. In subsequent years even complications that I assumed would never reverse have done so.

Within a year I had refined my insulin and diet regimen to the point that I had essentially normal blood sugars around the clock. After years of chronic fatigue and debilitating complications, almost overnight I started to gain weight, and at last I was able to build muscle as readily as nondiabetics. People commented that my gray complexion was gone. Although I had been conditioned to fear eating fats and protein — the medical professionals told me that was guaranteed to send my cholesterol level through the roof — it turned out that my cholesterol had by then not only dropped but was at the low end of the normal range.

My insulin requirements dropped to about one-third of what they had been a year earlier. With the subsequent development of human insulin, my dosage dropped to less than one-sixth of the original.

In a TV movie, my doctor would try other patients on the same diet, they'd have the same results, and within a few hundred frames of film the whole of the American Diabetes Association (ADA) would have its own epiphany and do an about-face. Diabetic complications would evaporate, and within a few years every diabetic would be doing what I had done. Someone would win a Nobel Prize for medicine.

Of course, that's not the way the world works. I found myself in a quandary: everything I had been taught was wrong, and I could prove it — but nobody was listening. My doctor wasn't interested, so I wrote a paper on my findings and even distributed it to many medical professionals, but it was uniformly ignored. All of my attempts to publish my discoveries in medical journals were met with ridicule by the editors. Nineteen seventy-six — the year of my death — came and went. I believed the only way I could beat the establishment was to join it, so at age forty-five I went to medical school.

When I finished medical school and went into practice, I assumed that I would be treating type 1 diabetics like myself. Again I did not quite have a crystal ball. The vast majority of my patients were type 2 diabetics, people whose problem was not that they couldn't gain weight, but that they couldn't lose it. I found, however, that the program that I had been continuously developing for people like me worked equally well for them.

Now, nearly forty years since I became certain my days were numbered, I am doing fine. I did not cure my diabetes, but I have what a cure will provide: normalized blood sugars. It's ironic to think that if and when there is a cure for diabetes, I and those who have used my program will likely prove to be healthier than many of those who someday are cured.

If I had never had to study my disease and all the factors that contribute to it or alleviate it, I would never have discovered how damaging high blood sugar or high insulin levels can be. I might have remained one of those people wolfing down a muffin or bagel for breakfast or picking at the bread basket on the restaurant table. Even with diabetes, I've found much better health than many nondiabetics with carb-heavy diets, and you can too.

When I hear diabetics longing to "be normal" again, they're most often not talking about being healthy — they can have that, even with diabetes — but about not having to worry about what they eat. I don't worry about what I eat, I enjoy it. There are many things that you can eat — many foods you have probably been conditioned to fear as "heart-attack food" or are now confused about because of divergent views on what low carbohydrate really means. Based on years of self-experimentation, I can clear up that confusion.

As a general rule, I'm not a big fan of diet books. Most are based on a promise of weight loss that is never achieved. Some low-carbohydrate diet books cause their adherents to lose weight too quickly then gain it back, with the too-frequent result that they end up fatter and less healthy.

There is also the issue that nearly all the most successful diet books on the market are part of a larger marketing strategy: get people on your WOW diet and make compliance easiest if they buy WOW bars and WOW shakes and other WOW tie-in products. Some of these are little more than cheap junk food in high-priced packages, and I've rarely seen any that are truly low in carbohydrate. There's even a story that a bestselling low-carbohydrate diet "expert" changed the "ideal" percent of carbohydrate in the diet because otherwise the company could not get the bars to stick together properly. I am not selling bars and shakes. I have seen very few that would fit in a truly low carbohydrate diet. As you will discover, my definition of low-carb is considerably different from the popular perception.

Although you may not notice it, much of the "science" that underlies various diet programs is shoddy. Doctors — who should know better — toss around terms like "reactive hypoglycemia" without apparently any real understanding. It is all too easy to accept popular ideas at face value without ever really examining them in depth.

This is where I differ. For many years I accepted the medical orthodoxy, and it almost killed me. I've long had a saying: "What works, works." When a new idea comes along, if I think it will stand up to scrutiny, I'll try it out on myself. If it works, wonderful. If not, I discard it.

Whether you're overweight, obese, diabetic, or simply looking for the healthiest way of eating, there is no better diet than this one. When I prescribe this diet to my patients, what I am prescribing are parameters, within which patients can choose what to eat. Most diet books will lead you by the nose — one size fits all — unless the book has a gimmick to it, like metabolic or blood type or ethnic origin. Even then you are likely to be led by the nose.

With the Diabetes Diet you make the decisions on what you are going to eat and, within guidelines, how much.

With this book you will create your meal plan. It's simple, and I think you'll agree with me that being energetic, healthy, and slim are certainly preferable to lethargy, chronic pain, and a slow death — regardless of whether you have diabetes.

PART ONE

About the Diabetes Diet

1

Why a Low-Carb Diet Is the Only Answer for Diabetics

AND A VERY GOOD ANSWER FOR EVERYONE ELSE

In its March 30, 2001, edition, the respected journal *Science* published "The Soft Science of Dietary Fat," by Gary Taubes. The article was not in the strictest sense groundbreaking. It was almost more about the politics of diet than the science. For doctors like me who have been writing for decades about the dangers of a low-fat, high-carbohydrate diet and the benefits of a low-carbohydrate diet, Taubes's article was not so much news as a kind of vindication. What Taubes did was show in clear and convincing detail that there was precious little evidence to support the prevailing hypothesis: that high cholesterol levels and other indicators of cardiac and other disease risk were a consequence of dietary fat, and that dramatically reducing fat and substituting large amounts of carbohydrate would reverse those risk factors. It's a hypothesis that many people still cling to fervently, despite mounting evidence to the contrary. There never were, and still have never been, any studies supporting the notion that dietary fat is the killer it was for decades claimed to be. Taubes writes:

15

> Despite decades of research, it is still a debatable propo-
> sition whether the consumption of saturated fats above
> recommended levels . . . will increase the likelihood of
> untimely death. . . . Nor have hundreds of millions of
> dollars in trials managed to generate compelling evi-
> dence that healthy individuals can extend their lives by
> more than a few weeks, if that, by eating less fat.

There are, however, many special-interest groups deeply
vested in the high-carbohydrate, low-fat hypothesis.*

Because "The Soft Science" was published in a magazine that is well known and respected for its rigorous and
carefully researched reporting on science, and because the
article was well researched, well reasoned, and well sourced,
it was the catalyst for a tectonic cultural shift in attitudes on
diet — on what is good for you and what is not.

Taubes won the National Association of Science Writers 2001 Science in Society Journalism Award for his work,
but the real earthquake that set off the cultural shift was another article, also by him, that covered similar ground but
reached a vastly larger audience.

On Sunday, July 7, 2002, millions of New Yorkers and
other readers around the world woke up to the question,
posed on the cover of the *New York Times Magazine,*
"What If It's All Been a Big Fat Lie?" The cover showed a
photograph of a succulent, nicely marbled steak with a pat
of butter melting on top. The article inside convincingly explained that what most people have been told about carbohydrate, protein, and dietary fat is wrong.

---

*Links to Taubes's articles can be found on the Internet site for this
book, www.diabetes-book.com.

16

In 1997, when my book *Dr. Bernstein's Diabetes Solution* was published, a low-carbohydrate diet was still a fairly radical concept. (When I published the first version of my diet and treatment plan, in 1981, low-carb diets were absolutely on the fringe.) According to nearly all major media, fat was poison. It was making us overweight, clogging our blood vessels with cholesterol, killing us with heart disease, diabetes, and so on. Quite a number of "experts" maintained that so-called complex carbohydrates, such as whole grain breads, oats, and pasta, were the answer to nearly every dietary need.

What was happening then — Americans getting fatter, the incidence of diabetes increasing dramatically — kept happening, and it is still happening today.

Over the last several years, with the wide success of low-carb weight-loss plans such as the Atkins Diet, Sugar Busters, the South Beach Diet, and Protein Power, the once-heretical concept of a low-carbohydrate diet has moved from the fringe to the mainstream — despite the continuing protestation of many diet "experts." Alfred Lubrano, in the *Philadelphia Inquirer,* wrote on December 7, 2003:

> Avoiding bread, pasta and potatoes at what food experts say is an astonishing rate, many Americans are evangelically fixated on the low-carbohydrate dining espoused by diets such as Atkins and South Beach. Depending on the estimate, between nine million and 35 million people are following all or some of the tenets of a high-protein, low-carb eating regimen.*

---

*Http://www.philly.com/mld/inquirer/news/front/7430619.htm.

In the same article, Lubrano also writes: "Unlike *low-fat* and *low-calorie,* there are no government guidelines defining the term *low-carbohydrate.* The Grocery Manufacturers of America Inc. has petitioned the Food and Drug Administration to come up with a working definition, which food analysts say may happen early next year."

These diets have achieved widespread acceptance with readers and dieters if not with many old-school dietitians because they help people lose weight and lower several cardiac (and other disease) risk factors. We have now reached a flashpoint, and today low carb is a fad. A recent article by Candy Sagon in the *Washington Post,* "Low-Carb Crazed: Food Producers Scramble to Please a Nation Obsessed," included the following:

> The supermarket is rapidly filling with new low-carb products. . . . I tried low-carb Sara Lee white bread spread with Skippy "Carb Options" peanut butter. I grilled a burger and squirted on Heinz's One Carb Ketchup (regular ketchup has more sugar). I sucked down a low-carb Michelob Ultra and wished that I could try the new low-carb Tostitos Edge or Doritos Edge that Frito-Lay is test-marketing in Phoenix and promising to introduce nationally in May. Pasta is a big no-no on the Atkins plan . . . but trust the food industry to develop low-carb pasta (five kinds under various brand names including Mueller's), and saucemakers like Ragú to introduce a new low-carb pasta sauce. Since steak is big on a high-protein diet, Lawry's has a low-carb version of its steak sauce. And although the Girl Scouts haven't come out with a low-carb Thin Mints cookie, candymaker Russell Stover has introduced low-carb mint patties. Snapple and Tropicana . . .

now have new low-carb drinks made with the artificial sweetener sucralose.*

The author also describes so-called low-carbohydrate offerings at many fast food restaurants, including Burger King, Subway, Baja Fresh, Hardees, and Blimpies. McDonald's and Wendy's have also joined the parade.

It is a blessing that low-carbohydrate diets have gained widespread acceptance, and that a lot of people now have at least some idea (but likely not a very good one) about the role of insulin in building body fat.

It's a bit of a curse, however, that the diets have taken hold so suddenly, because fads tend to promote false and misleading information. I suspect that the largest percentage — if not 100 percent — of the products mentioned in the *Washington Post* article are not in fact low carb by my standards. Among the "experts" there is little agreement on what low carb *means,* and when you throw marketing mavens into the mix (the same people who slapped NO-FAT! claims on candy), things become even more oversimplified as the ka-ching of supermarket cash registers rings throughout the land.

A decade or two ago, people clambered aboard the low-fat bullet train like the station was on fire. Fat was bad, low fat was good. No fat was even better. Where people had been calorie counters in the past, they threw that out the window as the train was pulling out, and started pigging out on low-fat foods. If the label said low fat, the thinking apparently went, it was okay to eat as much as you liked. As long as you avoided the "heart-attack foods" like steak and

---

*January 28, 2004, page F01.

butter and sour cream, you could keep the no-fat potato. But in fact, the reverse was true.

Now there is the very real likelihood that we will start pigging out on so-called low-carb foods, thinking them virtuous while simultaneously having no idea why. (The grocery boutique Trader Joe's has begun a very significant low-carbohydrate campaign in its stores, providing a guide to the low-carbohydrate foods. They even have a significant stock of "no-carbohydrate" candies, which are sweetened with sugar alcohols rather than table sugar. In truth, because these contain alternate forms of sugar, they are not sugar free, despite the labeling laws.)

There is simply no question that a truly low carbohydrate diet — namely the one presented in these pages — is the solution for diabetics. Indeed, it's the solution to the obesity that plagues increasingly sedentary populations around the world.

HOW A LOW-CARB DIET WORKS

A low-carb diet is superior for one simple reason: if done according to the guidelines (in this case I am referring to the guidelines in this book), people don't get fat, or don't stay fat, even as they reach the years of the supposedly inevitable "middle-age spread." In addition, all of the indicators for disease that are supposedly controlled by a low-fat diet, such as triglycerides and LDL (or "bad") cholesterol, descend to normal or low-normal ranges in most people. It's been shown over and over again that slim (not underweight) people live longer than fat people, or even people who are just heavy.

The reason that a low-carb diet can help you become

or remain slim is tightly linked to the hormone insulin, which is the principal fat-building hormone. The process works like this: The lower the amount of fast-acting or concentrated carbohydrate you eat, the less significant is the increase of your blood sugar. The less significant the effect on your blood sugar, the less of the fat-building hormone insulin you will need (either injected or made by your body) to stabilize blood sugar. With less insulin at large in your bloodstream, fats you eat will not be stored but metabolized (you will literally pee them away as water or breathe them away as carbon dioxide). In addition, as blood sugars decrease, the efficiency of insulin increases, further minimizing insulin levels in your body, with the result that existing body fat will start to metabolize as well — it will, as they say, just melt away.

Besides playing a role in diseases that result from overweight and obesity, excessively high serum insulin levels are toxic to the body and carry a number of effects that reduce longevity. These include increased blood pressure and damage to the lining of the blood vessels, or endothelium. These effects increase the likelihood of heart attack, stroke, and atherosclerosis, in addition to other vascular difficulties.

In general, a low-carbohydrate diet provides the nutrients that people need without the excess carbohydrate that causes high blood sugars and requires high levels of insulin. In addition, protein, fat, and slow-acting carbohydrate, such as leafy and whole-plant vegetables and some kinds of root vegetables, tend to be broken down more slowly and continuously, so people who follow this diet tend to feel satisfied much longer after eating. It has also been shown that people on low-carbohydrate diets can consume more calories while losing the same amount of weight as those on simple restricted-calorie diets.

Although the diet I prescribe for my patients has been available to the public since the publication of my first book, *Diabetes: The Glucograf Method for Normalizing Blood Sugar,* in 1981, I never have published the diet separately until now. There are two reasons I have felt it necessary to do so.

First, as the number of diabetic, overweight, and obese people continues to increase, and as the popularity of low-carbohydrate diets increases, many dieters, frustrated with the failure of the dietary recommendations of the American Diabetes Association and the American Heart Association (AHA), are looking for an alternative. Surfing diabetes-related Web sites, discussion boards, and chat rooms, you'll see low carb everywhere — but you'll also see a lot of misconception as to what low carb means. As diabetics look for an alternative to the ADA and AHA recommendations, it's important that the advice be sound. *Dr. Bernstein's Diabetes Solution* is a comprehensive program for normalizing blood sugar and covers all the bases — medication, exercise, diet, blood sugar self-monitoring — but I hear over and over again about the diet portion: "Nobody *ever* told me that before." People who despaired of ever losing weight, ever having energy, ever being able to carry on a healthy sexual relationship, have said again and again that the diet was the main thing that helped them regain control of their lives. I've seen people shed 50 or more pounds in a few months and say they had never before felt in control of their appetites or their lives.

The second reason for this book is that because diabetes, obesity, and overweight are so closely intertwined, I have treated many nondiabetics — some who were in danger of becoming diabetic, others who just wanted to lose weight. I have seen them reverse their complications (which they had despite being "not diabetic"), shed enormous amounts of weight, and regain their health and energy.

I recently saw a man who weighed more than 400 pounds. Clinically speaking, he wasn't a diabetic. In working him up, I found that his blood sugar levels were indeed slightly elevated, although not as much as I had suspected, and that he already had about fifteen diabetic complications. Most doctors would say to this man, "Lose weight and let's keep an eye on those blood sugars." This is effectively shifting the burden to the patient and not providing medical care.

I treated him as though he already was a diabetic. My definition of diabetic is anyone with elevated blood sugars, relative to the mean of normal (or the average for the healthy, young, adult nondiabetic population). In all likelihood, however, even the mean of normal is questionable as a safe standard because of the way the general population eats. A recent study published in *Diabetes Care* showed that in the United States the mean of normal was an average blood sugar level of 95 mg/dl (milligrams of glucose per deciliter of blood). For what I see in slim, young adults, a mean of about 83 mg/dl is really normal.

What this demonstrates is that there are a lot of Americans walking around with elevated blood sugar levels, and over time, even if they haven't been clinically diagnosed as diabetic, they are at serious risk for developing the complications associated with diabetes. The diet in this book is not just a diabetes diet, it's a longevity diet, a disease-prevention diet, and a fitness diet. It is the reason that although I have a "fatal illness," I am healthier than many considerably younger people.

It is also the reason that the cardiac and kidney risk factors of the gentleman described above dropped significantly over the next few months and his weight is coming under control.

WHY THE DIABETES DIET IS SUPERIOR

It's arguable whether any of the low-carbohydrate diets in the bookstores today is ideal for nondiabetics. But I can say that none of them is ideal for diabetics. Most of them depend heavily on the glycemic index, which is a subjective rather than objective evaluation of the speed of the action of carbohydrate on blood sugar. What does that mean? Sugars and starches are all carbohydrate. The body breaks them down at different rates; for example, 10 grams of glucose is going to affect your blood sugar considerably more rapidly than 10 grams of carbohydrate in spinach. The glycemic index (which we will discuss in greater detail in Chapter 3) attempts to rank most common foods by this speed — and thus the rapidity of the subsequent requirement for insulin (either made by the body or injected). The glycemic index, for reasons we'll get into later, is at best flawed and misleading. Many foods that I advise you to avoid are perfectly acceptable on mainstream low-carb diets that use it as a guide.

The Diabetes Diet works better than typical low-carb regimens for other reasons as well. The first is that, *within the guidelines,* you eat what you want and like to eat, but there are no "treat days." Many low-carbohydrate diet plans ignore the reality that much of overweight and obesity is directly related to carbohydrate addiction and constant snacking. This may be because many dietitians and diet doctors really don't understand carbohydrate addiction, although the mechanism has been well documented (see page 135). Treat days are a little like having a smoker go all week without a cigarette and then saying, "Go ahead and have a cigarette on Saturday." My experience with my patients has demonstrated over and over that for people with a history of overeating "treats," it's much simpler just to give up the treats than to have the self-discipline to eat only one small portion of sweets or starches on a treat day. I have also found that when most people give up fast-acting carbohy-drate, their desire to snack, indeed, their *need* to snack, goes away too. And, of course, treat days and the resultant high blood sugars make no sense for diabetics.

The second notable difference between the structure of this diet and others is that there are no "phases" here. The amounts of carbohydrate that you ought to eat will remain essentially constant for life. For purposes of weight loss, or if you significantly increase or decrease your physical activ-ity, protein amounts can be adjusted, but that's about it. In that respect, this diet is much simpler to follow.

In most of the low-carb diets I know of, you begin on a highly restricted regimen and then, just as you start to lose weight nicely, you change your diet. You start to reintro-duce into your meal plan foods that tend to be high in fast-acting or concentrated carbohydrate. These diets often add the caveat that after phase one you will stop losing weight or slow your weight loss but you can stay on phase one for a longer period of time if you want to lose more.

There are a number of problems with this kind of phas-ing. A significant one is that if your weight loss is too fast — for instance, if you starve yourself — you're likely to get on the yo-yo diet roller coaster. Why? Your body can't make glucose from fat, so if you're starving yourself, your quick-weight-loss diet may reduce your stores of protein (after your body converts some to glucose) in addition to fat. Your protein stores are principally your muscle mass. If you lose 10 pounds, you may lose 5 pounds of muscle in addition to 5 pounds of fat. If and when you gain back 10 pounds (or more) — which is likely because you're starving — what you gain back will be mostly fat. You'll end up worse off than when you started.

Another result is that you will have decreased your sensitivity to insulin, because our ratio of fat to muscle mass is one of the main factors affecting insulin sensitivity. Decreased sensitivity to insulin, also called insulin resistance, means there will be more of this fat-building hormone in your bloodstream.

From the perspective of a diabetic, phasing makes achieving normalized blood sugars considerably more difficult, in part because you will likely need to make several adjustments to your medications. Medications for diabetes, in particular injectable insulin, must be carefully fine-tuned. We'll talk about this a little more in the next chapter.

Just as important is the issue of carbohydrate addiction. Most low-carb diets might as well add the caveat that after phase one, you're going to quit the diet because suddenly you're back to the same old stuff that got you into trouble in the first place.

My college classmate became obese after years of poor diet, which included carbohydrate addiction and a lot of snacking. Then, several years ago, he went on a low-carbohydrate diet and lost about 45 pounds over the course of a relatively short period. He looked great, felt great, had a whole new outlook and a whole new wardrobe. Then one evening he was at a party and "just had one" cracker. No problem, he thought. But it was the same as if he'd been a smoker who'd stopped and then just had one cigarette. It was impossible to stop at just one, and his diet never recovered. He gained back the weight he lost in almost no time. The consequence? He's in much poorer health than he was, and his lipid profile is back in the unhealthy range. His new wardrobe, his newfound health and energy, his whole new outlook — all of that is out the window.

The restricted phase of these diets also plays into the not very healthy view of diet as a continuum between sin and virtue. The fast-food chain Subway ran an ad campaign that exemplified this, with an actor doing something "sinful" but excusing it by saying, "It's okay, I had Subway for lunch." (Subway sandwiches, by the way, have no place in this diet, not even their new "low-carb" sandwiches — unless you throw away the bread.)

Gluttony is one of the seven deadly sins, and from that frame of reference, the tendency is to look at abstinence as virtue and at indulgence as vice. The phasing of diets (and the treats) creates an unfortunate dynamic of deprivation and reward. Get through boot camp, so to speak, and then you can relax. Just lose that 20 pounds so you can fit into your wedding dress or tuxedo and look good for the pictures, then gorge yourself on the honeymoon, because you've got a mate and don't have to look your very best anymore. This is not healthy thinking and not healthy dieting.

My aim is not to deprive you or starve you. The "reward" for the "virtue" of this diet is a healthy weight and overall health and longevity. In the end, you'll find it far more satisfying than the so-called yo-yo effect that phased diets regularly cause.

Finally, many people seem to equate low carbohydrate with high protein. That may be true of some diets, but not of this one. As noted previously, amounts of protein can be adjusted to suit individual needs, but I do not subscribe to the myth that as long as you aren't eating fast-acting carbohydrate there is no need to limit protein intake. A certain amount of protein does get converted to blood sugars by the body, and that will raise insulin levels and build fat. (Still, if you're going to overeat or binge, a 42-ounce steak is not as likely to lead to incessant snacking as a 42-ounce bag of corn chips.)

The idea here is to put yourself on a single regimen and then just stay with it. I provide guidelines, and the diet doesn't change much except in what you select to eat. Then depending on how rapidly you lose weight (or don't), and on any lifestyle changes (pregnancy, training for a marathon, or an injury that interrupts your regular exercise, for example), the amount of protein you consume may be changed. In that respect, there could hardly be a more reliable, simpler diet.

The wonderful recipes in this book have been created by a chef and restaurateur whose son is a type 1 diabetic. You could live off these innovative and creative dishes forever, but I encourage you to eat what you like and enjoy your eating within the guidelines. We have gourmet dishes that will have your friends or your mother-in-law asking for the recipe. We also have fast breakfasts for when you're on the go. So use the guidelines and the tools provided, and be healthy, feel great, and live long.

2

Some Basic Science Underlying the Diabetes Diet

A variety of physiological factors other than the food you eat can and will affect blood sugars. Some of these, such as exercise and insulin resistance, are obvious and well known. Others are rarely if ever addressed in diabetes diets, but they're crucial if you are to be successful in normalizing your blood sugars. Most of these are in some ways applicable to nondiabetics as well. The pages that follow contain simplified discussions of these phenomena, in order to get you jump-started. For those who want to know more, I've provided the page numbers in *Dr. Bernstein's Diabetes Solution* where further details can be found (all page number references are to the 2003 edition).

THE LAWS OF SMALL NUMBERS
(*Diabetes Solution*, page 99)

"Big inputs make big mistakes; small inputs make small mistakes" is an indispensable piece of wisdom for life as well as for diet.

Many biological and mechanical systems respond in a predictable way to small inputs but in a chaotic and considerably less predictable way to large inputs. As an example, think about traffic. Put a small number of cars and trucks on a given stretch of highway and traffic acts in a predictable fashion: you can maintain speed, enter and merge into open spaces, and exit with a minimum of danger. There's room for error. Double the number of cars and the risks don't just double, they increase geometrically. Triple or quadruple the number of cars and the unpredictability of a safe trip increases exponentially.

The name of the game for the diabetic in achieving blood sugar normalization is predictability. It's very difficult to use medications safely unless you can predict the effect they'll have. Nor can you normalize blood sugar unless you can predict the effects of what you're eating on your blood sugars.

If you can't accurately predict your blood sugar levels, then you can't accurately predict your needs for insulin or oral blood sugar–lowering agents.* If the kinds of foods you're eating give you consistently unpredictable blood sugar levels, then it will be impossible to normalize blood sugars.

For people who use insulin, the Laws of Small Numbers are absolutely crucial because when you inject insulin, not all of it reaches your bloodstream. The more insulin you use, the greater the level of uncertainty. An unpredictable portion of injected insulin is destroyed by the liver and the immune system. How and where you inject can affect ab-

---

*I only recommend two kinds of oral agents for treating diabetes — those that increase the body's sensitivity to insulin, or those that act like insulin without potential adverse effects. See page 224 of *Dr. Bernstein's Diabetes Solution,* 2003 edition.

sorption of the commonplace large doses as well. According to researchers at the University of Minnesota, a 20-unit injection in your arm will result in an average 39 percent variation in the amount that makes it into the bloodstream from one day to the next. Abdominal injections had a 29 percent average variation.

These are enormous variations. These numbers are averages, remember, so on any given day, your injection of the same amount could be twice or half as effective as the one on the day before. The larger your doses of insulin, the bigger the discrepancy. So if you eat large amounts of carbohydrate that you need to cover with large doses of insulin, your ability to predict your insulin needs is almost nil. If you inject 20 units of insulin at one time, a 29 percent variability will, *on average,* create a 6-unit discrepancy in your absorption (could be 8 units, could be 4). Since 1 unit lowers a typical 150-pound adult's blood sugar by 40 mg/dl, the result is, *on average,* a 240 mg/dl blood sugar uncertainty (40 mg/dl x 6 units). The good news is that at doses smaller than 7 insulin units for adults, the absorption uncertainty becomes negligible. This diet enables us to use smaller doses of insulin, keeping unpredictability in check.

Another Law of Small Numbers relates to the fact that in the United States, food manufacturers are permitted an error of plus or minus 20 percent when estimating carbohydrate content on product labels. For a customary 150-gram carbohydrate portion of pasta, this boils down to a typical blood sugar uncertainty of 150 mg/dl (5 mg/dl/gm x 150 gm x 20 percent). For 2 cups of salad containing a total of only 12 grams carbohydrate, the blood sugar uncertainty would be only plus or minus 12 mg/dl. The uncertainties in food value books may sometimes be double or quadruple those on labels, making high carb values even more risky.

31

Bottom line: observing the Laws of Small Numbers in counting carbs and, correspondingly, injecting insulin will help you get control of your diabetes or your weight.

DIMINISHED PHASE I INSULIN RESPONSE   (*Diabetes Solution*, page 89)

The normal blood insulin response to a meal comes in two phases. During the time between meals, your body stores up insulin in order to respond to the next meal. When you eat, phase I is the instant release of stored insulin in response to the "glucose challenge" of the meal you've started to eat, and it prevents a sharp rise in blood sugars. Phase II is slower and longer in duration, and consists of the release of insulin as your body is making it.

In type 1 diabetics both phases of blood insulin response are nonexistent. In type 2 diabetics the first phase is diminished or absent. This is one of the hallmarks of type 2, and the reason blood sugars can rise sharply shortly after beginning a meal. Intramuscular insulin injections approximate the phase II response, but there is no way, medically, to mimic the phase I response. Thus a low-carbohydrate diet, which requires less insulin, is absolutely essential for normalizing blood sugars.

GLUCONEOGENESIS (*Diabetes Solution*, page 90)

Gluconeogenesis is essentially Latin for "new creation of glucose." If you were a healthy nondiabetic and hadn't had a meal in 3 days, your blood sugar levels would probably still be essentially within a normal range. Why? The body can convert protein to glucose. This includes protein you eat, but also stored protein — as in your muscles and other tissues, which continually receive amino acids (the "building blocks" of protein) from and return them to the bloodstream. This constant exchange makes amino acids always available for conversion to glucose. So (to simplify) for the nondiabetic, if you haven't eaten, your body senses the drop in blood sugars and converts stored protein to glucose; meanwhile, the normal insulin response keeps blood sugars from going too high.

For the diabetic with a major insulin deficiency, the problem is that insulin response may not be enough to bring blood sugars back into line. So even though you haven't eaten, if you test your blood sugars you'll find they're high. In the old days, before insulin became available for injection, type 1 diabetics were said to melt away into sugar water.

In all likelihood, you won't be able to control this phenomenon by diet alone, particularly if you're a type 1 diabetic or a type 2 making too little insulin to offset your insulin resistance (see below). For type 2s, appropriate weight loss and vigorous exercise may be essential to improving your body's sensitivity to insulin.

THE DAWN PHENOMENON
(*Diabetes Solution*, page 91)

As you know, I'm a type 1 diabetic and no longer make any insulin at all. If I decide to eat absolutely nothing for 24 hours, I'll still need to inject a small amount of long-acting insulin in the morning to prevent gluconeogenesis over the next 18 hours.

If I check my blood sugars every few hours, they will be constant over that period.

At the end of 18 hours — roughly at bedtime — I'll need to inject more insulin to continue to prevent gluconeogenesis.

It would stand to reason that I should be able to inject the same amount to cover the next 18 hours. But that's not necessarily the case. If I did inject the same amount and arose more than 8½ hours after my bedtime shot, when I checked my morning blood sugar, I'd find that it had not remained constant — despite the same amount of long-acting insulin — but had risen significantly higher than it was at bedtime.

If I did the same thing a week later, I'd get the same results — an overnight rise in blood sugars. Why?

Although the mechanics of the Dawn Phenomenon aren't yet entirely clear, research suggests that the liver deactivates more circulating insulin — self-made or injected — during the early morning hours than at other times of the day. With inadequate circulating insulin to prevent gluconeogenesis, your blood sugars may be higher in the morning than they were at bedtime.* This isn't a problem for a nondiabetic, because a nondiabetic would just make more insulin.

Investigators have actually measured blood sugar every hour throughout the night under similar circumstances and have found that the entire blood sugar increase occurs about 8–10 hours after bedtime for most affected people.

---

*Having an alcoholic drink at bedtime can inhibit gluconeogenesis overnight, but not predictably.

The amount of the increase may vary from person to person. My increase is significant; someone else's may be negligible.

Though it is more apparent in type 1 diabetics, many type 2 diabetics also show signs of the Dawn Phenomenon. Later, when we discuss the diet guidelines, you'll note that the amount of carbohydrate I recommend for breakfast is half that of lunch and dinner. The reason is the Dawn Phenomenon.

DELAYED STOMACH-EMPTYING
(*Diabetes* Solution, page 343)

This condition has a chapter all its own in *Diabetes Solution,* and if you suspect you have it — or if you have been diagnosed with it — I urge you to read that chapter and learn as much as you can. I know three people who experienced daily episodes of unconsciousness and seizures from time to time after meals for several years before I met them and diagnosed this condition.

The medical name for delayed stomach-emptying is gastroparesis diabeticorum (Latin for the "weak or paralyzed stomach of diabetics"). Nerve damage from high blood sugars over a long period of time can result in the failure of the stomach to empty predictably. This means that for those with gastroparesis, the same meal can have different effects on blood sugars from one day to the next, depending on how rapidly or slowly it empties from the stomach. This makes predicting insulin requirements less than simple, but there are treatments that are effective for many diabetics with this condition.

INSULIN RESISTANCE CAUSED BY HIGH BLOOD SUGARS
(Diabetes Solution, page 94)

There are at least five causes of insulin resistance — inheritance, dehydration, infection, obesity, and high blood sugars. The higher blood sugars are, the less effective insulin is. Insulin resistance, at least for type 1 diabetics, occurs as blood sugar increases, and so elevated blood sugar should be corrected as soon as it's feasible. Delay will only permit it to rise higher. Because type 2s still produce some insulin, their bodies are more likely to correct the blood sugar rise.

THE CHINESE RESTAURANT EFFECT
(Diabetes Solution, page 95)

Years back, a patient asked me why her blood sugar jumped significantly every afternoon after she went swimming. I asked what she ate before the swim. "Nothing, just a freebie," she replied. As it turned out, the "freebie" was lettuce. When I asked her how much lettuce she was eating before her swims, she replied, "A head."

The small amount of digestible carbohydrate in lettuce should not by itself have caused her blood sugar jump, even considering the quantity she ate. The explanation lies in what I call the Chinese Restaurant Effect. Some Chinese restaurant meals contain large amounts of protein or slow-acting, low-carbohydrate foods, such as bean sprouts, bok choy, mushrooms, bamboo shoots, and water chestnuts, that can make you feel full.

During and after meals, the stomach empties a slurry of

food mixed with liquid into the small intestine. The liquid passes through the small intestine and is absorbed, mostly in the large intestine. The solids stretch the walls of the small intestine as they slowly pass through. Cells in the upper part of the small intestine release hormones that signal the pancreas to produce insulin when they're stretched. (The pancreas is the gland responsible for manufacturing, storing, and releasing insulin in the body.) Large meals cause greater stretching of the intestinal cells, which in turn will secrete proportionately larger amounts of these hormones.

A very small amount of insulin released by the pancreas can cause a large drop in blood sugar, and so the pancreas produces the less potent hormone glucagon to fine-tune the potential excess effect of the insulin. Glucagon acts to increase blood sugar.

The problem arises when the insulin-producing cells of your pancreas — the pancreatic beta cells — make little or no insulin. Glucagon is still produced, but adequate insulin is not available to offset its effect.

The first lesson here is: Don't stuff yourself. The second lesson is: There's no such thing as a freebie. Any solid food that you eat (even pebbles) can raise your blood sugar if you're diabetic. Trivial amounts, however, such as a small stick of celery, will have negligible effects.

THE HONEYMOON PERIOD
(*Diabetes Solution*, page 96)

At the time they are diagnosed, type 1 diabetics usually have experienced very high blood sugars that cause a host of unpleasant symptoms, such as weight loss, frequent urination, and severe thirst. These symptoms subside soon after treatment with injected insulin begins. After a few weeks many patients experience a dramatic reduction of insulin requirements, almost as if the diabetes were reversing. Blood sugars may become nearly normal, even with low insulin doses. This benign honeymoon period may last weeks, months, or even as long as a year. If your treatment is conventional, the honeymoon period eventually ends and the roller coaster of blood sugar swings ensues.

There are several hypotheses as to why conventional treatment won't let the honeymoon go on forever, but my experience with patients indicates that *with proper treatment* it can. Essential to this is a low-carbohydrate diet and normal blood sugars. This will help preserve whatever insulin-producing pancreatic beta cells you may have. (The same is true for type 2 diabetics. Beta cell burnout — the destruction of beta cells caused by excessive demands on the pancreas and by the toxic effect of high blood sugars upon beta cells — can be avoided, halted, and in some cases reversed if you get on the *Diabetes Solution* program and get your blood sugars normalized.)

The bottom line here is that if you have been newly diagnosed and are experiencing a blood sugar honeymoon, get with the *Diabetes Solution* program as soon as possible.

3

Essential Guidelines
for the Diabetes Diet

In the days before low-carb diets began their tremendous upswing in popularity, it was difficult for people to overcome resistance to the idea of restricting carbohydrate in their diet. That job has become easier in the last few years, but at the same time there is still a tremendous amount of confusion about what carbohydrate foods ought to be emphasized and what ought to be restricted.

You'll hear people talk incessantly about complex and simple carbohydrates, but those are very loose categories and change depending on who is doing the talking. For our purposes, "good" carbohydrate is slow-acting and not concentrated. In keeping with the Laws of Small Numbers, good carbohydrate has a small impact on your blood sugar. Examples are whole-plant vegetables, leafy greens, mushrooms, and many others. These are foods that are either very difficult or impossible for the body to break down into glucose. Cellulose is a major component of vegetable foods — in addition, it's also a major component of wood — and while it is technically a carbohydrate, humans lack the enzymes to break it down. Cellulose is beneficial in a number of different ways, but most significant for our purposes is that cellulose "dilutes" the digestible carbohydrate and thereby slows its absorption. (Interestingly, eating fat with carbohydrate can further slow the digestion of carbohydrate, so if you have butter on your string beans or oil and vinegar on your green salad, this addition of fat will slow the absorption of the digestible carbohydrate.)

"Bad" carbohydrate is fast-acting or concentrated carbohydrate. This includes everything from straight table sugar to so-called complex carbohydrates like potatoes, carrots, whole grain bread, and peas (and many others).

SOME WORDS ABOUT CALORIES, AND WHY YOU OUGHT TO IGNORE THE GLYCEMIC INDEX

One of the most popular concepts with respect to low-carb diets is the glycemic index. The idea that underlies the glycemic index is that foods can be evaluated for their effect on blood sugars, in much the same way that they can be evaluated for their caloric content. The glycemic index (or GI) is the cornerstone of some of the bestselling low-carb diets. Even if you have no idea what it is, it's still likely that you've heard of it.

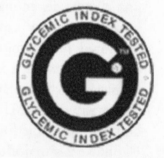

In Australia there is even a nonprofit organization that offers its imprimatur (a bit like the Underwriters Laboratory seal or the Good Housekeeping seal) to foods that "meet

The glycemic index seal. If it comes to the United States, ignore it.

specific nutritional criteria and have had their GI measured using the approved method. High, medium, and low GI foods are eligible."

It sounds like an elegant idea. Pure glucose equals 100. Mashed potatoes rate a 90 (depending on the group doing the testing). Table sugar rates a 70. As with a lot of seemingly elegant ideas, however, the reality is far more complex, just as the measure of calories is more complex than it appears.

What a Calorie Really Is

You probably can't even remember the first time you heard of a calorie. But you know what it is, right? Or do you? Well, let's look at calories for a moment.

A calorie is an objective measure of energy — specifically, it's the energy given off as oxygen rapidly oxidizes foodstuffs (that is, when they are burned). One calorie is the amount of energy it takes to raise the temperature of 1 milliliter of water 1 degree Celsius. Our bodies burn energy, but in a much slower and different way than does fire. So when you read a food label and it says 100 calories, this is not a direct measure of anything the food actually does in your body, or of how much it will affect your waistline, but a measure of how much the burning food in a testing laboratory raised the temperature of a specific amount of water. There is a margin for error allowed in food labeling, of course, so the stated measure is not absolutely exact.

By this measure, 1 gram of dietary fat contains 9 calories, 1 gram of dietary protein contains 4 calories, and 1 gram of dietary carbohydrate also contains 4 calories. A gram of alcohol contains 7 calories.

This all sounds very simple and straightforward, but in

41

fact it is not. Consider that if you, like the calorimeter used to measure the calories in food, burned all of the calories in the food you ate, you would rarely need to move your bowels. Consider also that a two-by-four would burn and heat up the water in a calorimeter very nicely, but the calories it contains would be almost entirely from cellulose, the same indigestible fiber making up much of the carbohydrate content of, for example, most vegetables.

Fat, while it will keep your lamp burning, is less straightforward than carbohydrate. Fat plays various and significant roles all over the body — in the brain and in the makeup of hormones and cell membranes throughout — and the body expends more energy extracting the energy from dietary fat than it does extracting the energy from carbohydrate. Recent evidence has shown that while fat may gross 9 calories per gram, the net available for metabolism is closer to something like 5 calories a gram.

Protein is similarly complicated. Meats, for instance, contain not just protein but also indigestible gristle, water, and fat; beans or other vegetable sources of protein may "trap" some of the protein in indigestible fiber; and of course protein can be used by the body in the form of amino acids or may be slowly converted to glucose. In fact, generally speaking, there are only about 6 *grams* of real protein in an *ounce* of a protein food, even though by weight there are 28.47 grams in a U.S. ounce. The Diabetes Diet uses this 6 grams per ounce figure in converting grams of protein (as you might find them listed in food value tables or on nutrition labels) to ounces of a protein food. Chapter 5, "Customizing the Diet," shows you how this works.

So the bottom line is that despite our ability to measure the caloric content of foods objectively, what we're getting is a rough estimate at best.

What's Wrong with the Glycemic Index

The glycemic index seeks to measure the impact that particular foods have on blood sugar. It's my opinion that there is simply no way to determine objectively — without measuring an individual's blood sugars — how any given food at any given time is going to behave in any given individual.

The notion of the glycemic index was first conceived of by Dr. David Jenkins around 1980 in attempting to find foods that were appropriate for diabetics. The index numbers you may have seen are derived from graphs of the averages that particular foods have on both diabetics and nondiabetics. Since glucose is the blood sugar, dietary glucose is the standard against which other foods are measured, and rates a GI of 100. Whole wheat bread rates a 70 on one scale, while it comes in at 99 on another. Whole grain pasta rates a 45 or a 53, depending — again — on the group who did the testing.

The baseline 100 number represents the area under the curve of a graph depicting a rise in blood sugar over 2 hours from eating a particular number of grams of glucose. You take another carbohydrate food — whole wheat bread or pasta, for example — containing an equal amount of carbohydrate, then plot the 2-hour curve of the resulting blood sugar rise after eating it. The glycemic index number comes from dividing the area under the test food's curve by the area under the glucose curve and then multiplying by 100 to get percent.

Dr. Jenkins defined the glycemic index of a carbohydrate food in terms of how its curve related to that of the glucose curve. If a food has a glycemic index of 50, then the area beneath its curve is 50 percent of the area beneath the glucose curve.

So what's wrong with that?

Well, as it turns out, a lot of things.

As attractive as it may seem, the glycemic index, unlike the measurement of calories, seeks to quantify something much less hard and fast. Instead of measuring the heat released by burning a food in a laboratory, the glycemic index plots the average of a considerably more variable series of chemical and physiologic reactions that occur within the human body.

When you eat, the digestive process begins pretty much as soon as food hits your saliva. How digestible a food may be depends not just on your body and its ability to produce enzymes and hormones, but also on how the food was processed (cooked, chopped, ground, pureed, etc.). How you react to foods depends on a host of factors, from your own physiology to the combinations of foods you are eating. Fats, for example, tend to slow down digestion.

The only way to measure the real effect of foods on blood sugar is to feed people the foods, then frequently measure blood sugar for a given period of time, then average the results.

For a type 1 diabetic like me, it's easy to see the effect that, say, a bagel has on my blood sugar. Since I make no insulin, I have no built-in mechanism to automatically bring down the ensuing blood sugar surge. The surge for a non-diabetic man of similar height, weight, and age is going to be much less. My experience with my patients has been that a food that can raise my blood sugar significantly might have a similar but not exact effect on the blood sugar of another type 1 diabetic. It will not have the same effect on a type 2 diabetic — nor will the effect be the same from one type 2 to another. Many things besides the foods we eat can affect blood sugar — everything from insulin resistance to adrenaline surges and exercise to infection to the quantity of what we eat (don't forget the Chinese Restaurant Effect) — especially for the diabetic.

While the glycemic index reflects only the 2-hour period after eating a food, in reality it typically takes 5 hours to fully digest the carbohydrate portion of a meal (in the absence of gastroparesis). This discrepancy has been justified by the claim that "while digestion and absorption may take 5 hours or more, most of the blood glucose fluctuation takes place in the first 2 hours. That's where big differences between foods become apparent and where damage might be done to the body. Small differences seen after 2–3 hours are not of major clinical significance."*

On the surface this position doesn't seem particularly unreasonable — but it reflects a basic ignorance of the impact that issues "not of major clinical significance" can have on diabetics. Having lived with this disease for nearly sixty years, I know intimately how things that seem of small significance to the nondiabetic clinician can in reality completely defeat efforts to normalize blood sugars. The same food that makes my blood sugar rise dramatically may have little or no effect on that of one of my patients who still makes considerable insulin.

Because the GI is an average, true numbers vary considerably from one person to another, from one time to another, and from one study to another. But even if we accept it as a given that the glycemic index is an accurate reflection of the effect that carbohydrate foods have on blood sugar —

---

*Jennie Brand-Miller, author of *The New Glucose Revolution*, responding to a question from medical writer Rick Mendosa on www.mendosa.com/bernstein.htm.

which is simply not the case — there is still the issue of interpretation. What is low, medium, or high?

I would say that if a food is going to be classified as low, then it must not provoke a sharp increase in blood sugar levels. It should allow you to adhere to the Laws of Small Numbers and keep your need for insulin — whether injected or made by your body — to the minimum.

I seem to be in the minority here — not an unusual position for me. A lot of well-meaning dietitians and diabetes educators now use the glycemic index to recommend foods that are "low" but in reality are completely inappropriate in a sensible blood sugar normalization regimen. According to www.glycemicindex.com, low, medium, and high glycemic indices are as follows:

- Low = 55 or lower
- Medium = 56–69
- High = 70 or above

My own experience is that a vast number of foods that are rated low by this definition will cause considerable blood sugar elevations in diabetics. In addition, these foods will impede blood sugar normalization in diabetics and contribute to weight gain or prevent weight loss in nondiabetics.

The carbohydrate foods that I recommend in the ensuing pages — salads and selected vegetables — typically have glycemic indices less than one-quarter that of the "low" threshold above.

I recommend that you ignore the glycemic index, because in the final analysis it is no more helpful than the old calorie system of weight loss. Calorie counts give us a rough idea of the energy available from a particular food, and the old idea was that you could lose weight if you ate less and burned more calories. So you would guesstimate your daily caloric burn based on your height, weight, age, and so forth. Then you could count calories and eat fewer than you burned. That always sounded good on paper, but my experience is that it never really worked.*

Using the glycemic index, by comparison, tells us what? Its original intent was to find foods appropriate for diabetics. Again, however, there is the question of interpretation. The apparent conclusion of the popular press on low-carbohydrate diets is that you can eat your fill of low-GI foods and still lose weight. As long as we eat foods with a GI of 55 or lower, the thinking goes, the pounds will just melt away, diabetes will fall into line, and all will be well with the health of the population. I wish it were so.

And now, added to the concept of the glycemic index is the "glycemic load," which was developed by Dr. Walter Willett. The idea behind the glycemic load (GL) is that the glycemic index of a food doesn't tell you enough. (Which I would support.) The glycemic index tells you *how fast* the carbohydrate in a particular food turns to sugar, but it doesn't tell you *how much* carbohydrate is actually in a

---

*The beta oxidation (or "burning") of fat by the body requires the action of an enzyme called insulin-sensitive lipase. This enzyme is turned off by insulin. Eating carbohydrate obliges the body of a nondiabetic to make insulin in proportion to the amount consumed and obliges many diabetics to inject insulin to prevent blood sugar elevation. When insulin levels go up, fat oxidation therefore goes down, and since insulin is also the fat-storage hormone, dietary fat is stored. Furthermore, insulin signals the liver to convert the carbon backbone of carbohydrates (glucose) to saturated fat, which then appears in the blood as triglycerides, which are subsequently stored. So calories of fat are handled much differently on a low-carbohydrate diet than on a high-carbohydrate diet. Recent studies on humans eating equivalent amounts of fat show that those eating more carbs store more fat.

serving of that food. The blood sugar effect of a "serving" of a very dense food like a potato is likely to differ considerably from the effect of a serving of a less dense food such as popcorn. The glycemic load, which takes carbohydrate density and serving size into account, is supposed to give you a better view of the overall burden the food you eat places on your body.

Unless you're very clever and keep a calculator and a book of indices with you at all times, this seems to me unnecessarily complex and labor intensive. Are you going to sit down at a restaurant with your book of the glycemic index and have the waiter go over the gram count of the foods on the menu? Will you do the calculations when you open up a recipe book?

I think it's a great idea to know what you eat. But I also think that all this calculation is too much like the old system of "exchanges" — "Well, since a slice of bread has a glycemic load of X and this other food has a glycemic load of X and a half, if I just eat two-thirds of the slice of bread — no, wait a minute. . . ."

In addition, the glycemic load theory assigns foods different numbers than the glycemic index, so there is always the potential for confusing them.

Keeping It Simple

There are no complicated formulas or calculations in the Diabetes Diet. In the following pages I will show you the foods that you ought to emphasize in your diet and the foods you ought to eliminate.

There are two kinds of carbohydrate, fast-acting (concentrated) and slow-acting (dilute). Eat a limited amount of the slow (for which I provide guidelines in the pages to come) and eliminate the fast/concentrated. That's about as complicated as it gets. Next time you're in a restaurant or at a buffet, you can look at the foods that are available and have a very good idea what you should eat and how much — without a calculator and an index.

The guidelines are simple and are provided so that you can use your own common sense to judge what's acceptable in your diet and what's not. Before long, you'll find it all very easy.

NO-NO FOODS: SAY GOOD-BYE TO THE REAL HEART-ATTACK FOODS

If you have tried weighing glycemic load against glycemic index, or other similarly murky concepts, in order to figure out what and how to eat — forget it. It doesn't have to be that arcane or difficult, and you don't need a math degree.

In the pages that follow are several lists. Most important is the list of common foods that contain fast-acting carbohydrate and should be eliminated from your diet. This includes virtually all grain products. Pure bran (hard to find) is the exception. So-called complex carbohydrate like brown rice, whole wheat flour in "sugar-free" cookies, pasta (whether al dente or cooked to mush), breakfast cereals (including noble oatmeal), corn, and other grain products are transformed into glucose so rapidly that in terms of their effect on blood sugar and insulin requirements, they are just like table sugar.

Other foods — ones that contain very small amounts of simple sugars — fall into a middle area. A single stick of chewing gum or tablespoon of salad dressing that contains 1

In or Out? A Simple Test

Here's a really simple and objective way for you to tell if a food is in or out. Sometimes you'll find yourself at a restaurant, hotel, or reception where you have no idea whether the food you're about to be served has fast-acting, concentrated carbohydrate in it. Your waiter probably has little idea, or will tell you what he thinks you want to hear, so don't even ask. I've found that the easiest way to make certain is to use Clinistix or Diastix test strips. These are made for testing for the presence of glucose in urine and are available at most pharmacies. I find them handy for testing for sugar or starch in foods.

Say you want to find out if a soup, salad dressing, or sauce has sugar or flour in it. Put a small amount in your mouth, mix it well with saliva (saliva is essential to the test because it breaks down table sugar and starches to glucose), then spit a tiny bit onto the test strip. You can tell by the color it turns approximately how much, if any, fast-acting carbohydrate it has in it. The absence of color change on the test strip indicates no glucose. A very slight color change may be acceptable for foods you'll eat in small amounts. You can also use this method with solid foods, but you'll have to chew the food first.

This is a method that can be very useful for finding and eliminating fast-acting or concentrated carbohydrate from your diet. Carry a pack of the sticks with you and when in doubt, test.

gram of carbohydrate is not going to wreak havoc on the ability of most diabetic adults to control blood sugar. But if you're the kind of person who — like the old commercial said — can't eat just one, but chain-chews gum or likes to have a major league baseball–sized wad going, you should probably avoid chewing gum (although small amounts of "sugar-free" chewing gum may help the digestion of those with delayed stomach-emptying; see *Diabetes Solution,* Chapter 22). If you eat salad only because you love the dressing, then you'll have to use your judgment and your blood sugar profiles* and possibly switch to a vinaigrette or dressing that leaves out sugars entirely (such as the Blue Cheese Dressing or the Parmesan Dip in the recipe section of this book).

Powdered Artificial Sweeteners

If you're wary that artificial sweeteners might contain chemicals that could cause ill effects (cyclamates, remember, were banned in the United States because lab rats got cancer after eating the human equivalent of truckloads), I'd recommend first that you weigh the theoretical risk of lab rats and cancer against the very real, exhaustively researched ill effects caused by sugar. So far the harm resulting from the use of sugar is of considerably more concern, particularly for diabetics, than risks associated with artificial sweeteners.

If you want to research artificial sweeteners and find which you like best and which seem of lowest risk, I encourage you to do so. If you feel that you don't need to use sweeteners, then by all means avoid them.

---

*See *Diabetes Solution,* especially Chapters 4 and 5.

Food Count Bibles

Here are a few of the books of food values that can be helpful in figuring out your meal plan.

- *The NutriBase Complete Book of Food Counts* (Avery, 2001). $14.95 (paperback). My favorite.
- *Bowes & Church's Food Values of Portions Commonly Used,* 18th ed., Jean A. T. Pennington and Judith S. Douglass (Lippincott Williams & Wilkins, 2004). $49.95 (plastic comb bound).
- *The Complete Book of Food Counts,* 5th ed., Corinne T. Netzer (Dell, 2000). $7.50 (paperback).

Personally, I have seen no ill effects from them, and I find them quite pleasant as additions to desserts like my no-pie pumpkin pie, which is just unsweetened pumpkin pie filling mixed with some cinnamon and stevia or another sweetener. Without the cinnamon and sweetener, in my opinion, the pumpkin is about as tasty as Kleenex. With it, it's a pleasant treat.

If you've rarely used artificial sweeteners and think you won't care for them, let me assure you that it really doesn't take long to get used to them.

At this writing, there are several artificial sweeteners available from different manufacturers under different names, and some, such as Equal and Sweet'n Low, are multiple sweeteners sold under the same brand name in different packaging. Here, to simplify your shopping, are acceptable sweeteners currently or soon to be available:

- Saccharin tablets or liquid (Sweet'n Low)
- Aspartame tablets (Equal, NutraSweet)
- Acesulfame-K (Sunette, The Sweet One) — Not yet available in tablets or liquid form.
- Stevia powder or liquid — Has not been approved in the European Union.
- Sucralose (Splenda) — This is actually a sugar (the *-ose* ending indicates sugar), but one that the body does not recognize and does not break down. It is not yet available in the United States in tablet or liquid form, except in things like Da Vinci syrups. Demand is such, however, that a liquid version may soon be available in the United States.
- Neotame — Newly approved by the U.S. Food and Drug Administration (FDA) but so far only being marketed to manufacturers.
- Cyclamate tablets and liquid — Not yet available in the United States, but sold in Canada under the name Sugar Twin.

These sweeteners vary in their availability and cost. All can be effectively used to satisfy a sweet tooth without, for the most part, affecting blood sugars.

Note that the only acceptable powder on the list above is stevia. Other powders contain an additive to increase bulk. That additive happens to be sugar, most often in the form of glucose or maltodextrin or both, and though the packet label will claim it's 0 carb, or 0 calories, that's only because the serving size comes in under the FDA radar — that is, 0.9 gram of dextrose doesn't constitute a "significant amount." But I have learned from experience that it will rapidly raise blood sugar a significant amount if you consume a few packets.

Bottom line: Don't use powdered sweeteners except stevia. If you are the kind of person who likes your coffee or tea sweet, then carry a container of the tablets of your choice — or stevia powder — with you in your purse or pocket.

A new "natural artificial" sweetener, called tagatose, will soon be available under the brand name Naturlose from Spherix, Inc., in the United States. Derived from milk, it's claimed to be 92 percent as sweet as sugar and said to have similar bulk, with no aftertaste and no effect on blood sugars. Whether it really does have no effect on blood sugar remains to be seen. It is being marketed as requiring no added glucose or maltodextrin to bulk it up, so if it is indeed sold in powdered form without added sugars, it may be a valuable addition to the arsenal.

In many cases, what manufacturers and nutritionists and doctors call "no effect on blood sugars" or "negligible effect" has significant enough effect to make blood sugar control more difficult.

Another new artificial sweetener, neotame, is being sold as an additive by the makers of NutraSweet. It is supposedly 8,000 times as sweet as table sugar. Its use as a food additive should pose no problems, but if it becomes available as a powder over the counter, it will probably be mixed with a sugar as in the instances cited above.

So-Called Diet Foods and Sugar-Free Foods

In the recent past, food labeling laws in the United States have permitted products to be called sugar-free if they do not contain common table sugar (sucrose). Such labeling requirements have the effect of allowing manufacturers to perpetuate a myth that sugars that are not sucrose (table sugar) are not sugars, which is nonsense. Still, it fools a lot of people. I've been in doctors' offices that have candy dishes full of "sugar-free" hard candies especially for their diabetic patients. If you read labels, you can often find out what kind of stealth sugar is in the product, but individually wrapped candies may not have labels.

Here is a partial list of stealth sugars. All of these will raise your blood sugar. Keep in mind that sugars (and carbohydrate) tend to end in *–ose* (as in lactose), while sugar alcohols end in *–ol* (as in sorbitol).

Stealth Sugars

carob	lactose	saccharose
corn syrup	levulose	sorbitol
dextrin	maltitol	sorghum
dextrose	maltodextrin	treacle
dulcitol	maltose	turbinado
fructose	mannitol	xylitol
glucose	mannose	xylose
honey	molasses	

Some, such as sorbitol and fructose, raise blood sugar more slowly than glucose but still too much to prevent blood sugar rises after eating in people with diabetes.

Other "diet" foods contain stealth sugars or large amounts of rapid-acting carbohydrate, or even both. A sugar-free cookie, for example, is virtually 100 percent rapid-acting carbohydrate (flour), so that even if it contains none of the stealth sugars, a small quantity would easily cause rapid blood sugar elevation.

There are exceptions:

- Most diet sodas are fine, although there are glaring exceptions. Sugar-free Slice contains 40 percent "natural fruit juice." Bottom line: check the nutrition facts label and look for a goose egg — 0 — under carbohydrate. (A great thing about diet drinks: if you spill them, they're not sticky.)
- Sugar-free Jell-O brand gelatin desserts are also fine, but again you have to check the label. The ready-to-eat variety is currently sugar-free, but the powdered mix contains maltodextrin.
- Da Vinci brand sugar-free syrups (see page 88) use Splenda and are good for all sorts of uses, from flavoring and sweetening coffee to making sugar-free soft drinks (mix with sparkling water) or adding to vinegar and oil to customize a salad dressing.

All of these "exceptions" are made without sugar of any kind.

Candy, Including "Sugar-Free" Brands

Even a tiny candy like a SweeTart can raise blood sugars (indeed, I have used them to counteract low blood sugar episodes). A stealth sweetener like sorbitol tastes about a third as sweet as sugar, so candy makers use three times as much. As a consequence, it can eventually bring on about three times the blood sugar rise of table sugar. However, because of the recent low-carb fad, new candies and candy bars have come on the market that are said to be carbohydrate-free. With these, the bottom line is that you must read labels and, when in doubt, use Clinistix and check blood sugars. It's worth mentioning again, however, that the Clinistix/Diastix method will not detect sorbitol and other stealth sugars.

Nutrition Facts	Amount/Serving		% DV	Amount/Serving		% DV
	Total Fat	8 g	12%	Total Carbs.	14 g	5%
Serving Size: 25 g	Sat. Fat	5 g	25%	Fiber	3 g	12%
4 Servings per bar	Cholest.	0 mg		Sugars	0 g	
Calories 110	Sodium	7 mg	0%	Maltitol	11 g	
(5.5% DV)	Protein	1 g				

* Percent Daily value (DV) are based on a 2,000 calories diet.
Not a significant source of Vitamin A, Vitamin C, Calcium and Iron.

★ ★ ★ ★ ★ ★ ★ ★
Total Carbs: 14 g
Poly Alcohols (Maltitol): 11 g
Fiber: 3 g
NET IMPACT CARBS: 0 g
★ ★ ★ ★ ★ ★ ★ ★
Polyols: (Sugar Alcohols)

(Maltitol) has been omitted as its conversion requires little or no insulin and does not cause an appreciable increase in serum glucose levels.

INGREDIENTS: Maltitol, Cocoa Mass, Cocoa Butter, Inulin, Emulsifier (Soya Lecithin), Flavor.

Look for our other low carb products . . . we're sure you'll find a favorite

This is the nutrition facts label of a CarbSafe candy bar. The claim made on the label that sugar alcohol requires little or no insulin and will not cause an appreciable rise in blood sugars is fiction. The "net impact carbs" claim is deceptive.

Honey and Fructose

Honey and fructose (fruit sugar) have been touted as useful to diabetics because they are "natural" and more complex than table sugar. Glucose is *the* most natural of the sugars, since it is present in all plants and all but one known species of animal. Both honey and fructose will raise blood sugar far more rapidly than medication or phase II insulin response can effectively counter. Both are concentrated carbohydrates, so avoid them.

Desserts and Pastries

With the exception of products marked "carbohydrate — 0" on the nutrition label, virtually every food commonly used for desserts will raise blood sugar too much and too fast. This is not just because of sugar but also because flour, milk, and other components of desserts are very high in rapid-acting carbohydrate. You will find dessert recipes in this book that provide truly slow-acting, low-carbohydrate ways of satisfying your sweet tooth. Avoid the fast-acting

No-No's in a Nutshell

Here is a concise list of foods to avoid that are discussed in this chapter. You may want to copy it and keep it with you until you have the concept in hand.

Sweets and Sweeteners

- Powdered sweeteners (other than stevia)
- Candies, especially so-called sugar-free types
- Honey and fructose
- Most "diet" and "sugar-free" foods (except sugar-free Jell-O gelatin when the label doesn't mention maltodextrin, and diet sodas that do not contain fruit juices or list other carbohydrate on the label)
- Desserts (except Jell-O gelatin without maltodextrin — no more than ½ cup per serving) and pastries: cakes, cookies, pies, tarts, etc.
- Foods containing, as a significant ingredient, products whose names end in *-ol* or *-ose* (dextrose, glucose, lactose, mannitol, mannose, sorbitol, sucrose, xylitol, xylose, etc.), except cellulose; also, corn syrup, molasses, maltodextrin, etc.

Sweet or Starchy Vegetables

- Beans: chili beans, chickpeas, lima beans, lentils, sweet peas, etc. (string beans, snow peas, and green or red bell and chili peppers, which are mostly cellulose, are okay, as are limited amounts of many soybean products)

- Beets
- Carrots
- Corn
- Onions and tomatoes, except in small amounts
- Packaged creamed spinach containing flour
- Parsnips
- Potatoes
- Cooked tomatoes, tomato paste, and tomato sauce
- Winter squash
- Yellow bell peppers

Fruit and Juices
- All fruits (except avocados)
- All juices (including tomato and vegetable juices — except, for some people, in a Bloody Mary)

Certain Dairy Products
- Milk
- Sweetened, low-fat, and skim-milk yogurts
- Cottage cheese (except in very small amounts)
- Powdered milk substitutes and coffee lighteners
- Canned milk concentrate

Grains and Grain Products
- Wheat, rye, barley, corn, "whole grain" products, and lesser-known "alternative" grains, such as kasha, quinoa, and sorghum

continued on next page

Grains and Grain Products (*continued*)
- White, brown, wild rice, or rice cakes
- Pasta
- Breakfast cereal — including oatmeal of any variety
- Pancakes and waffles
- Bread, crackers, and other flour products

carbohydrate you'll find in most pies, cakes, and frozen desserts. Low-fat products are often the worst offenders.

Bread and Crackers

One average slice of white, rye, or whole wheat bread contains 12 or more grams carbohydrate. "Thin" or "lite" breads are usually cut at half the thickness of standard bread slices and therefore contain half the fast-acting, concentrated carbohydrate, but they are still unacceptable. So-called high-protein breads contain only a small percentage of their calories as protein and are not significantly reduced in carbohydrate unless they are thinly cut. Virtually all breads contain unacceptable levels of fast-acting carbohydrate, so it's best to avoid bread and crackers in general. There are some bran crackers that are acceptable because virtually all of their carbohydrate is indigestible fiber (see page 83).

Some diabetics with delayed stomach-emptying can include a slice of thin bread or one to two small crackers as part of their diet, but the rest of us experience very rapid in-

Prepared Foods
- Most commercially prepared soups
- Most packaged "health foods"
- Snack foods (virtually anything that comes wrapped in cellophane, including nuts*)
- Balsamic vinegar (compared to wine vinegar, white vinegar, or cider vinegar, balsamic contains considerable sugar)

creases of blood sugar after eating any grain product. This includes health food store grains, such as barley, kasha, oats, sorghum, and quinoa.

Rice and Pasta

Both pasta (when cooked al dente) and wild rice (not a true rice but actually another grain) are claimed by some nutrition authorities to raise blood sugar quite slowly. This is not true, as you can confirm by checking your blood sugar or trying the Clinistix/Diastix test. Like wild rice and pasta, white and brown rice also raise blood sugar quite rapidly for diabetics and should be avoided. The same is true of rice cakes. Al dente pasta is often touted as being "low" on the

---

*Even though some nuts are relatively low in carbohydrate, it's very difficult, for instance, to have a snack of just four macadamia nuts. That said, there are recipes in this book that use nuts — for example, the toasted nuts in the Cream of Artichoke Soup are only a small part of a larger recipe and add a little crunch and texture.

glycemic index scale because some of the grain isn't thoroughly cooked and therefore (the reasoning goes) acts more slowly on blood sugars. But it doesn't act slowly enough, which is further proof that the glycemic index is best ignored by diabetics. Avoid rice and pasta — whether al dente or boiled to mush.

Breakfast Cereals

Most cold cereals, like snack foods, are virtually 100 percent carbohydrate, even those claiming to be "high protein." Many have so much sugar, you might as well just eat candy. Even bran flakes are mostly flour. If you've been eating bran to improve bowel function, you can substitute psyllium husks powder, which is entirely indigestible fiber. Use only the sugar-free variety of Metamucil or other such products. (You can get the husks powder at a health food store and mix with water. If you don't care for the texture or taste, you can drink it mixed in diet soda. Some health food stores also have it in capsules, but you have to make sure you have plenty of water.) You can also make your own cereal from pure bran if you can find it in a health-food store.

Oatmeal, according to some low-carb diet books, has little effect on blood sugars. This could not be further from the truth. Breakfast cereals, cooked or cold, even in small servings, make blood sugar control impossible.

Snack Foods

One of the reasons many of my new patients are overweight or obese is that they snack incessantly. A few cookies here, a bag of chips or popcorn there, a candy bar or a couple of handfuls of little crackers — pretty soon you're on your way to overweight and obesity. These foods are virtually all carbohydrate and frequently have added sugar of one variety or another. Some nuts (macadamia, for example) are relatively low in carbohydrate, but who can sit down and eat only four? If you can, fine. Otherwise, it's best to avoid snacking entirely. Indeed, if you're an overweight snacker who eats for "recreation," you will likely find that shortly after beginning the Diabetes Diet, your need to snack will disappear. (See "Comfort Foods and Carbohydrate Addiction," page 135.)

Protein and Diet Bars

Although drugstore and grocery shelves are full of bars that claim to be "protein bars," frequently as meal substitutes, most are really nothing more than candy bars with "healthy" packaging. The FDA recently analyzed twenty different brands and found that all but two contained much more carbohydrate than stated on the labels. These were removed from the marketplace, but many more remain. This is another case showing that when it sounds too good to be true, it probably isn't true. Most protein bars associated with well-known diets have unacceptable levels of carbohydrate. There are plenty of so-called diet products whose main ingredient is sugar.

Avoid protein or diet bars as meal substitutes unless you are absolutely certain they have virtually no carbohydrate and no stealth sugar.

Milk

Milk contains a considerable amount of the simple sugar lactose and will rapidly raise blood sugar. Skim milk contains the most lactose per ounce; heavy cream has the least.

Although 1 or 2 teaspoons of milk in a cup of coffee will not significantly affect blood sugar, a few tablespoons will make a considerable difference to most of us. Cream, which you have probably been instructed to avoid, is okay. One tablespoon has only 0.5 gram of carbohydrate, and it tastes much better than substitutes and provides much better "lightening power."

Nondairy creamers, liquid or powder, contain relatively rapid acting sugars and should be avoided if you use more than a teaspoonful at a time or drink more than 1 cup of coffee at a meal. A coffee lightener worth considering is WestSoy brand soymilk, which is sold in health food stores and many supermarkets throughout the United States. Although several WestSoy flavors are marketed, only the one marked 100% Organic Unsweetened is unsweetened. The plain, unflavored variety claims only 5 grams of carbohydrate per 8-ounce serving. Other unsweetened and unflavored brands, such as Vitasoy and Yu Natural, are available in various parts of the country. One catch — soymilk curdles in very hot coffee or tea.

Here's a tip. If you drink coffee or tea at work and like it lightened, and if you share a common refrigerator with your coworkers, you probably find that when you bring in a pint of milk or half and half, it magically disappears. But your coworkers are probably conditioned to fear fat, so if you bring in a container of heavy cream, it will stay unmolested in the refrigerator — and it contains much less carbohydrate per serving.

Fruits and Fruit Juices

Most fruit juices have as much or nearly as much sugar and other fast-acting carbohydrate as regular soft drinks and will act dramatically on blood sugar levels. If you doubt this, you can prove it with a few experiments with blood sugar measurements. Some fruits and juices, despite their bitterness (for example, grapefruit and lemon) contain considerable amounts of simple sugars.

Learning to avoid juices used to be a big sacrifice for many of my patients, but it's increasingly accepted, thanks to the popularity of low-carb diets. Eliminating fruits as well, however, is a different matter. Most of us are accustomed to the idea that fruits and vegetables are a good thing, period. Most of what we commonly think of as fruit has a less rapid effect than juice on blood sugar, but fruits still cause an unacceptably large blood sugar rise. Some people fear that they will lose important nutrients by eliminating fruit, but that shouldn't be a worry. I haven't eaten fruit in more than thirty years, and I haven't suffered in any respect. Nutrients found in fruits are also present in the vegetables you can safely eat.

Most of us think of sweet fruits when we refer to fruit — apples, oranges, and bananas — all of which you should avoid. There are, however, a number of true biological fruits (the part of certain plants that contains pulp and seeds) that are just fine for the diabetic and the overweight or obese person trying to lose weight. These include summer squash, cucumbers (including many types of pickle), eggplant, bell peppers (green and red only), chili peppers, and avocado. These tend to have large amounts of cellulose, an indigestible fiber, rather than fast-acting carbohydrate, and they do contain vitamins and other essential nutrients.

In addition to being tasty and versatile, they can also promote digestive health for some people. It's worth noting that cellulose, found in vegetables and fruits, is essentially the same fiber that makes up much of the shady elm on the corner. It has indigestible calories your body won't metabolize. People don't have the enzymes necessary to break down cellulose, so it passes right through the digestive system without affecting blood sugars — so long as we don't eat excessive amounts that provoke the Chinese Restaurant Effect (page 36).

Vegetables

Just as some fruits are acceptable — some biological fruits, mentioned above — some vegetables are best avoided.

Beets. Like most other sweet-tasting vegetables, beets are loaded with sugar. Sugar beets are a source of table sugar.

Carrots. After cooking, carrots taste sweeter and appear to raise blood sugar much more rapidly than when raw. This probably relates to the breakdown of complex carbohydrates into simpler sugars by heat. Even raw carrots can be slowly converted to glucose and should be avoided. If, however, you are served a salad with a few carrot shavings on top for decoration, don't bother to remove them. The amount is insignificant, just like a teaspoon of milk.

Corn. Not a vegetable at all but a grain. Nearly all of the corn grown in the United States is used for two main purposes. One is the production of sweeteners. Most of the sugar in Pepsi-Cola, for example, comes from corn. The other major purpose is animal feed, e.g., fattening up hogs, cattle, and chickens. Corn for consumption by people, as a "vegetable" or in snack foods, comes in third. Diabetics should avoid eating corn, whether popped, cooked, or in chips — even 1 gram of corn (a couple of kernels of pop-corn) will rapidly raise my blood sugar by about 5 mg/dl.

Potatoes. In a steak-and-potato meal, it's the potato that's the heart-attack food. For diabetics, cooked potatoes raise blood sugar almost as fast as pure glucose, even though they may not taste sweet. Giving up potatoes in all their variety can seem a big sacrifice for many people, but it will also make a big difference in your blood sugars and your ability to lose weight and keep it off.

This book has a fabulous recipe for Mashed Cauli-flower that makes a very good substitute for mashed potatoes. The Parmesan-Crusted Zucchini slices could substitute nicely for home fries.

Tomatoes, tomato paste, and tomato sauce. Tomatoes, as you probably know, are actually a fruit, not a vegetable, and as with citrus fruits, their tang can conceal just how sweet they are. The prolonged cooking necessary for the preparation of tomato sauces releases a lot of glucose, and you would do well to avoid them. If you're at someone's home for dinner and are served meat or fish covered with tomato sauce, just scrape it off. The small amount that might remain should not significantly affect your blood sugar. If you are having them uncooked in salad, limit yourself to one slice or a single cherry tomato per cup of salad. (See page 258 for a low-carbohydrate, tomato-free, Italian-Style Red Sauce that can be good over, say, a broiled, sautéed, or grilled chicken breast or veal scaloppine.) Onions fall into this same category — despite some sharp flavor, they're quite sweet, some varieties sweeter than others. There are other vegetables in the allium family that can be substituted, although in smaller quantities, such as shallots and elephant garlic. A small amount of chopped onion (1 tablespoon) contains only 1 gram of carbohydrate and can readily be added to an omelet without adverse consequences.

Commercially Prepared Soups

Believe it or not, most commercial soups marketed in this country can be as loaded with added sugar as a soft drink. The taste of the sugar is frequently masked by other flavors — spices, herbs, and particularly salt. Even if there were no added sugar, the prolonged cooking of vegetables can break the special glucose bonds in the cellulose of slow-acting carbohydrates, turning them into glucose. As you know from above, the amount of carbohydrate claimed on a nutrition facts label can vary considerably from what's actually in the product. Add to that the common inclusion of potatoes, barley, corn, rice, and other unacceptable foods in soups, and you have a product that you will generally want to avoid. There are still some commercial soup possibilities that fit into our scheme (see page 79).

Health Foods

Of the hundreds of packaged food products that you see on the shelves of the average health food store, perhaps 1 percent are low in carbohydrate. Many are sweetened, usually with honey or other so-called natural sugars. Indeed, many natural foods can be very high in carbohydrate. Since the health food industry shuns artificial (nonsugar) sweeteners like saccharin or aspartame, if a food tastes sweet, it probably contains a sugar. If it isn't honey or fructose, then it may be another stealth sugar, such as sorbitol or maltitol. A few "health foods" are unsweetened and low in carbohydrate. Some of these are listed in the next chapter.

FAST FACTS ON WHAT TO EAT AND WHAT TO AVOID

Here is a summary of the kinds of foods you will want to avoid in order to maintain control over your blood sugar. Some of them are no-brainers, but others may surprise you. Many foods recommended by well-known low-carbohydrate diets as "low glycemic index" are too high in carbohydrate to make blood sugar control feasible. These are general categories, so some foods in the categories may be okay, but you will need to read labels carefully. When in doubt, check your blood sugar and use the Clinistix/Diastix method (see page 50) for checking the "sugar integrity" of the labels. This method will not detect sorbitol and other stealth sugars. If you need a "cheat sheet" to help you remember what's okay, make a copy of pages 75–94 and keep it with you. You might also want to copy the No-No list on pages 58–61.

Candy, Including "Sugar-Free" Brands

Even so-called sugar-free candies have lots of stealth sugars that will raise blood sugar. Some newer candies — ZCarb candy bars claim 0 carbohydrate — and others that may come on the market as the low-carbohydrate fad heats up might be acceptable. Unfortunately, most no- or low-carb brands misstate carbohydrate content, even though this is illegal.
BOTTOM LINE: **Avoid candies.**

Honey and Fructose

Touted as "natural" sugars, both are high in fast-acting carbohydrate.

BOTTOM LINE: **Avoid honey and fructose and any foods that contain them.**

Desserts and Pastries

Most are completely out, especially those that claim "low fat." On restaurant menus, dessert fruit cups may seem benign in comparison to Death by Chocolate, or crème brûlée, but avoid them (see Fruits and Fruit Juices, below). There are desserts in the recipe section of this book that are in step with the guidelines, plus other ways to satisfy a sweet tooth that won't significantly affect blood sugar.

BOTTOM LINE: **Avoid desserts that contain fruit, flour, sugar, or anything that ends in *-ol* or *-ose.***

Bread and Crackers

Among my patients only some of those with delayed stomach-emptying can eat a slice of bread without significant, immediate impact on blood sugar. The only brands of crackers I have found acceptable are those that are almost entirely fiber (see "Bran Crackers," page 83).

BOTTOM LINE: **Avoid both, even so-called high-protein bread.**

Rice and Pasta

Bestselling low-carb diets claim that al dente pasta is low or close to low in the glycemic index, and tout brown or wild rice. At this writing, nothing in this category will help you lose weight, avoid gaining it, or maintain normal blood sugars.

BOTTOM LINE: **Avoid everything in this category, including rice cakes.**

Breakfast Cereals

Some high-profile low-carb diets recommend particular cooked cereals, such as oatmeal. I know of no commercially available breakfast cereal, hot or cold, that will further your ability to normalize your blood sugars, even those that are "high protein." BOTTOM LINE: **Avoid all cereals.**

Snack Foods

This is an extraordinarily broad category, but it comprises mostly foods that are high in fast-acting carbohydrate. Most of my obese patients have problems here because they start out as incessant snackers, which fuels carbohydrate addiction. BOTTOM LINE: **There are really no acceptable snacks for diabetics other than sugar-free Jell-O without maltodextrin.**

Protein and Diet Bars

Even a protein bar or diet bar that is manufactured specifically to complement a low-carbohydrate diet is likely to be high in fast-acting carbohydrate. These products are best avoided; most are just candy bars with a high price tag and a fancy wrapper. BOTTOM LINE: **Avoid protein and diet bars even if they claim zero carbohydrate on the label, as virtually all such claims are deceptive.**

Milk

Milk's main purpose in the great scheme of things is to deliver healthy nutrients packed with fat and sugar to nursing infants, whether humans or other mammals. Skim milk is highest in lactose, or milk sugar; heavy cream is lowest. A small amount of milk in coffee (2 teaspoons) is acceptable; larger amounts are not. BOTTOM LINE: **Heavy cream or a very low carbohydrate soy alternative is best in your coffee or tea.**

Fruits and Fruit Juices

Most of the foods we commonly think of as fruits — oranges, peaches, bananas, grapes — are too high in fast-acting carbohydrate to make blood sugar control feasible. The juices of these are little more than sugar water.

BOTTOM LINE: **Avoid all fruits and fruit juices.**

Vegetables

Vegetables = Virtue. Actually, this is mostly true, except "vegetable" is a category more than a definition, and there are vegetables, mostly root variety — potatoes, beets, carrots — that are too high in fast-acting carbohydrate to be acceptable. Others that we think of as vegetables, such as tomatoes, are actually fruits.

BOTTOM LINE: **Avoid most root or tuber varieties (potatoes, beets, and carrots) and seed varieties (peas, most beans). Enjoy whole-plant or leaf vegetables.**

Commercially Prepared Soups

Unless the soup is a broth or consommé, it's almost impossible to know — even from the label — how high in carbohydrate it is.

BOTTOM LINE: **Make your own soups (the Italian Wedding Soup and Cream of Artichoke Soup recipes in this book are wonderful) or use bouillons or consommés labeled as having less than 2 grams of carbohydrate per serving.**

Health Foods

Very few so-called health foods are low in fast-acting carbohydrate. That may be changing, but to be sure, you should check labels, check blood sugars, and use the Clinistix/Diastix method.

BOTTOM LINE: **As with protein and diet bars, avoid most so-called health foods.**

4

So What's Low Carb?

Good question. In the days when I first developed this diet, virtually all of the carbohydrate foods I had been told were fine to eat made blood sugar control impossible, so I had to figure it out on my own. While something like the glycemic index rates carbohydrates at various levels, I have just two — carbohydrate that will make blood sugar control difficult or impossible, and that which makes it easy. This is a lot simpler than indexing or loading or exchanging — and unlike all those other methods of analyzing carb contents, it works.

The following pages contain an overview of the foods I eat and recommend to my patients. Please remember that with the exception of the no-calorie beverages (including the many different kinds of bottled waters that have no added carbohydrate) and moderate portions (half a cup) of sugar-free Jell-O without maltodextrin, there are no "freebies." Virtually everything you eat will affect blood sugar if you eat enough of it — remember the Chinese Restaurant Effect. So if you get that "once I start eating it, I just can't stop" feeling with a particular food, you should obviously avoid it altogether.

You may discover foods I've never heard of that in small amounts have a negligible effect on blood sugar. And there may be things that in small amounts do not affect your blood sugar that do affect mine. You should feel free to include them in your meal plan, but check your blood sugar every half hour for a few hours before assuming that they are benign.

FOODS FOR TRULY LOW CARB LIVING

Vegetables

Name ten vegetables you've eaten in the last 3 days. I'll bet most people can't. No wonder the FDA now requires that grain products have folic acid added. The sad reality is that people are more likely to eat grain products than green products. Folic acid, which derives its common name from the word *foliage* (its real name is pteroylglutamic acid), is plentiful enough in whole-plant and leafy green vegetables that we really shouldn't need to depend on supplements and treated foods. In addition, greens are a great source of bioavailable calcium, or calcium that the body can easily absorb. Most vegetables, other than those listed in the No-No list with a high level of fast-acting carbohydrate, are fine. Other vegetables to avoid would include those that fail the Clinistix/Diastix test.

As a rule of thumb, ⅔ cup of cooked vegetable, ¼ cup mashed cooked vegetable (depending on the density of the vegetable), or a cup of mixed salad acts upon blood sugar as if it contains about 6 grams of carbohydrate. Cooked vegetables tend to raise blood sugar more rapidly than raw vegetables because cooking makes them more digestible and converts some of the cellulose to glucose. As a general rule, more cooked vegetables will fit into a measuring cup than raw vegetables, particularly leafy vegetables. If you've ever sautéed spinach, you know that a skillet heaping with raw leaves will give you less than half a skillet of cooked spinach.

If you have diabetes, it's wise to keep daily records of your blood sugar and to note on your self-measurements how your favorite vegetables (or, for that matter, any food) affect your blood sugar. (See page 111 for an example of the GLUCOGRAF II data sheets I and my patients use to keep track of blood sugars.)

Raw vegetables can present digestive problems to people who experience delayed stomach-emptying. As noted before, if you have delayed stomach-emptying, also called gastroparesis, or if you think you might, the complete guide to dealing with it is in Chapter 22 of *Dr. Bernstein's Diabetes Solution.*

Of the vegetables listed on the facing page (the list is by no means exhaustive), 1 cup of raw and ⅔ cup of cooked vegetable (¼ cup if mashed) acts on blood sugar as if it contains about 6 grams of carbohydrate.

In addition to the foods on The List, keep the following in mind:

- Onions are high in carbohydrate and should only be used in small amounts for flavoring. You'll notice that most of the recipes in this book use shallots instead (shallots are from the same family as onion

**The List:
Really Good — and Good for You —
Low-Carbohydrate Vegetables**

Remember, as a rule of thumb, 1 cup of raw vegetable or ⅔ cup cooked vegetable (¼ cup if mashed) has approximately the same effect on blood sugar as 6 grams of carbohydrate.

artichokes
asparagus
bamboo shoots
beet greens
bell peppers (green
    and red only, no
    yellow)
bok choy (chinese
    cabbage)
broccoli
brussels sprouts
cabbage
cauliflower
celery
celery root (celeriac)
collard greens
daikon radish
dandelion greens
eggplant
endive
escarole
hearts of palm

kohlrabi
mushrooms
mustard greens
okra
patty pan squash
pumpkin
radicchio
rhubarb
sauerkraut
scallions
snow peas
spaghetti squash
spinach
string beans
summer squash
turnip greens
turnips
water chestnuts
watercress
zucchini
zucchini flowers

and garlic — the allium family — with a flavor sort
of halfway between the two). They — and chives —
pack a lot of flavor in small amounts.

- One-half medium avocado contains about 6 grams
  of carbohydrate.
- One cup mixed green salad without carrots and with
  a single slice of tomato or onion has about the same
  impact on blood sugars as 6 grams of carbohydrate.
- One-quarter cup mashed, cooked vegetable acts as if
  it contains about 6 grams of carbohydrate.

Meat, Fish, Fowl, Seafood, and Eggs

These foods are usually the major sources of calories in the
meal plans of my patients, and they are where you can make
most of the adjustments to your own plan so that you feel
satisfied. While meat and eggs have until recently been dietary pariahs, my personal observations and recent research
implicate carbohydrates rather than dietary fat in the heart
disease and abnormal blood lipid profiles of diabetics and
even of nondiabetics. If you are frightened of these foods,
you can restrict them, but depriving yourself will be unlikely to provide you any health benefit. Egg yolks, by the
way, are a major source of the nutrient lutein, which is beneficial to the retina of the eye. Organic eggs contain large
amounts of omega-3 fatty acids, which are good for your
arteries.

In some of the post-Atkins low-carbohydrate diets, there
has been an emphasis on "good" fats. Barry Sears, author of
The Zone, is a big proponent of the good-fat theory. I know
him, and I've tried out his theory with a few of my patients,
but I didn't see it change any part of their lipid profiles.

Tofu, and Soybean Substitutes for Bacon, Sausage, Hamburger, Fish, Chicken, and Steak

About half the calories in these products come from supposedly benevolent vegetable fats, and the balance from varying amounts of protein and slow-acting carbohydrate. They are easy to cook in a skillet or microwave. Protein and carbohydrate content should be read from the labels and counted in your meal plan (see Chapter 6 for details). The principal value of these foods is for people who are vegetarian or want to avoid red meat. Health food stores stock many of these products, and so do a growing number of supermarkets.

Certain Commercially Prepared and Homemade Soups

Although most commercial and homemade soups contain large amounts of simple sugars, you can easily learn how to buy or prepare low- or zero-carbohydrate soups. Many but not all packaged bouillon preparations have no added sugar and only small amounts of carbohydrate. Check the labels or use the Clinistix/Diastix test. Plain consommé or broth in some restaurants may (rarely) be prepared without sugar. Again, check with Clinistix/Diastix.

Homemade soups, cooked without vegetables, can be made very tasty if they are concentrated. If you have a no-carbohydrate broth recipe you find appealing, try making it with half the water, or try reducing it considerably to make it richer. Herbs and spices, which have negligible amounts of carbohydrate, are great for adding flavor — and they also have been shown to contain many different kinds of beneficial phytochemicals, or nutrients found in plant foods.

(See also "Mustard, Pepper, Salt, Spices, Herbs," below.) Clam broth (not chowder) is usually very low in carbohydrate. In the United States you can also buy clam juices (*not* Clamato), which contain only about 2 grams of carbohydrate in 3 fluid ounces. The clam chowder recipe in this book is delicious.

Campbell's canned beef bouillon and consommé contain only 1 gram carbohydrate per serving. College Inn canned chicken broth contains no carbohydrate. Most bouillon cubes are also low in carbohydrate. Read the labels.

Cheese, Butter, Margarine, and Cream

Most cheeses (other than cottage cheese; see below) contain approximately equal amounts of protein and fat and small amounts of carbohydrate, and you'll have to figure the carbohydrate and protein into your meal plan. For people who want (unwisely, from a health standpoint) to avoid animal fats, there are some special soybean cheeses, which are not very tasty, and there's hemp cheese. Cheese is an excellent source of calcium. Generally speaking, every ounce of whole-milk cheese contains approximately 1 gram carbohydrate and 6 grams of protein (which is equivalent to 1 ounce of other protein foods). There are exceptions to this; some Swiss cheese, for example, contains slightly more carbohydrate, and Gruyère contains virtually none. Generally speaking, where dairy products are concerned, the lower the fat, the higher the sugar lactose, with skim-milk cheeses containing the most lactose and the least fat, and butter containing no lactose and the most fat.

Cheese is made from fermented milk, a process in which most or all of the sugar is converted to carbon dioxide and water. Cottage cheese is only partly fermented and so still has a fair amount of lactose, so it should be avoided except in very small amounts, say about 2 tablespoons. Dry-curd cottage cheese is sugar-free but may be hard to find. It is also known as farmer's cheese and baker's cheese. It has very little flavor.

Neither butter nor margarine will, in my experience, affect blood sugar significantly, and they shouldn't be a problem as far as weight is concerned if you're not consuming a lot of carbohydrate along with them. One tablespoon of cream has only 0.5 gram carbohydrate — it would take 8 tablespoons to raise my blood sugar 20 mg/dl.

The cheese puffs I like to make are low in carbohydrate and can be used instead of bread to make sandwiches (see the Cheese Puff Sandwich recipe on page 172).

Yogurt

Although personally I don't enjoy yogurt, many of my patients feel they cannot survive without it. For our purposes plain whole-milk yogurt, unflavored, unsweetened, and without fruit, is a reasonable food. A full 8-ounce container of plain, Erivan brand, unflavored whole-milk yogurt contains only 11 grams of carbohydrate and 2 ounces of protein. You can even throw in some chopped vegetables and not exceed your 12-gram lunch carbohydrate limit (see the following chapter); some Middle Eastern and Indian dishes combine unsweetened yogurt with cucumbers, for example.

Do not use nonfat yogurt. The carbohydrate goes up to 17 grams in an 8-ounce container of unflavored nonfat yogurt.

Yogurt can be flavored with cinnamon, with Da Vinci

brand syrups (see page 88), or with baking flavor extracts such as vanilla liquid. It can be sweetened with stevia liquid or powder, dissolved Equal or Splenda tablets, or liquid saccharin. Erivan brand yogurt is available at health food stores throughout the United States. If you read labels, you may find brands similarly low in carbohydrate in your supermarket; two such brands are Stonyfield Farm and Brown Cow Farm. Be sure to use only the whole-milk versions and not the low-fat.

Soymilk

There are many soy products that can be used in our diet plan, and soymilk is no exception. It's a satisfactory lightener for coffee and tea, and one of my patients adds a small amount to diet sodas. Others drink it as a beverage, either straight or with added flavoring such as those mentioned for yogurt. Personally, I find the taste too bland to drink without flavoring, and I would probably prefer cream diluted with water. When used in small amounts (up to 2 tablespoons), soymilk need not be figured into the meal plan.

As noted in the No-No foods section, of the many brands of soymilk on the market, WestSoy offers the only unsweetened one I've been able to find, although other unsweetened brands are available in various parts of the country.

Soybean Flour

If you want to try baking with soybean flour, you'll find a neat solution to the pastry restriction in this diet. One ounce of full-fat soybean flour (about ¼ cup) contains about 7.5 grams of slow-acting carbohydrate and about 1 ounce of protein. You could make chicken pies, tuna pies, and even sugar-free Jell-O pies or pumpkin pies. Just remember to include the carbohydrate and protein contents in your meal plan.

Soybean flour usually must be blended with egg to form a batter suitable for breads, cakes, and the like. Creating a blend that works requires either experience or experimentation.

Bran Crackers

Of the dozens of different crackers that I have seen in health food stores and supermarkets, I have found only three brands that are truly low in carbohydrate.

- GG Scandinavian Bran Crispbread, produced by G. Gundersen Larvik A/S, Larvik, Norway (distributed in the United States by Cel-Ent, Inc., Box 1173, Beaufort, SC 29901, fax only, 843-524-9444). Each 9-gram slice contains about 3 grams of digestible carbohydrate. If this product is not available locally, you can order it directly from the importer or via the Web at www.ggbrancrispbread.com. One case contains thirty 4-ounce packages. They are also available from Trotta's Pharmacy, 877-987-6882.
- Bran-a-Crisp, produced by Saetre A/S, N1411, Kolbotn, Norway (distributed in the United States by Interbrands, Inc., 3300 N.E. 164th Street, FF3, Ridgefield, WA 98642). Each 8.3-gram cracker con-

tains about 4 grams of digestible carbohydrate. Bran-a-Crisp may be ordered directly from Interbrands, Inc., by phone or fax if you cannot find it locally. Phone 877-679-3552 or fax 360-574-3574. The Web site www.branacrisp.com will take you to on-line wholesalers and retailers, or you can order from Trotta's Pharmacy. This product is also available in some food markets as Fiber Rich bran crackers.

- Wasa Fiber Rye. These crackers are available in most supermarkets in the United States and in some other countries. One cracker contains about 5 grams of di-gestible carbohydrate. Many of my patients feel that this is the tastiest of these three products. Other Wasa brand crackers contain more carbohydrate.

Although some people eat these plain, to me they taste like cardboard without a spread or some other kind of flavoring. My preference is to enjoy them with chive-flavored cream cheese or butter. Crumbling two GG crispbreads (6 grams carbohydrate) into a bowl and covering them with water plus a tablespoon or two of cream can create bran cracker cereal. Add some Equal or Splenda tablets (dissolved in a bit of hot water) or some liquid stevia or saccharin and perhaps a baking flavor extract (fruit flavor, butter flavor, etc.), or one of the Da Vinci brand sugar-free syrups.

If eaten in excessive amounts, bran crackers can cause diarrhea. They should be eaten with liquid. They are not recommended for people with gastroparesis (delayed stomach-emptying), since the bran fibers can form a plug that blocks the outlet of the stomach. The small amount of digestible carbohydrate in these crackers is very slow to raise blood sugar. They are great for people who want a substitute for toast at breakfast.

NOTE: In the United States, labeling regulations require that fiber be listed as carbohydrate. There are different kinds of fiber, and they all behave differently. My rule of thumb is to deduct *half* of the stated grams of fiber from the stated grams of carbohydrate to get a general idea of how the listed carbohydrate will affect your blood sugars. Remember the Chinese Restaurant Effect. Even a product that is 100 percent fiber can raise blood sugar.

Toasted Nori

When my friend and fellow diabetic Kanji Ishikawa sent me a beautifully decorated canister from Japan, I was most impressed and intrigued. You can imagine my dismay when I removed the cover and found seaweed. My dismay was only temporary, however. I reluctantly opened one of the cellophane envelopes and pulled out a tissue-thin slice. My first nibble was quite a surprise — it was delicious. When consumed in small amounts, I found, it had virtually no effect upon blood sugar. Once addicted, I combed the health food stores searching for more. Most of the seaweed I tried tasted like salty tissue paper. Eventually, a patient explained to me that Kanji's seaweed is a special kind called toasted nori. It contains small amounts of additional ingredients that include soybeans, rice, barley, and red pepper. It is available at most health food stores, and is a very tasty snack. Five or six slices at a time have had no effect upon my blood sugar. The Clinistix/Diastix test showed no glucose after chewing. A standard slice usually measures 1 x 3 inches and weighs about 0.3 gram. Since the product contains about 40 percent carbohydrate, each strip will have only 0.12 gram carbohydrate. You can weigh larger sheets of toasted nori in order to estimate their carbohydrate content.

Artificial Sweeteners

Using artificial sweeteners other than "to taste" can be a little tricky. Such products can range from 30 times as sweet as sugar (cyclamate) to 8,000 times (neotame). Some break down in cooking, such as aspartame, which should be added after cooking or used only with cold food or drink. And some break down partially — Splenda retains 90 percent of its sweetness. Since none have the bulk of table sugar, in their powdered form they often are bulked up, frequently with dextrose (glucose) or maltodextrin, which are other sugars.

Some have an aftertaste, but sensitivity to it seems to vary from person to person. I like stevia, but you may find saccharin more appealing. Many people who cook with artificial sweeteners recommend blending them with saccharin to keep costs down.

Some desserts or treats are easy to make to taste, but others, particularly anything you're investing time in or that requires elegant presentation, really requires a level of predictability. When I make my pumpkin pie filling dessert with cinnamon and stevia, I do it to taste — I put the ingredients together and add stevia until its sweetness suits my palate.

The best advice I can give is that if you have a sweet tooth, use the rules of thumb presented below, and experiment. Until you are certain you have repeatable results, have some of the sweetener handy when you serve your treat in case it doesn't quite live up to your mouthwatering expectations. (The wavy equal sign ≈ means "approximately equal to.")

Aspartame. Equal tablets are said to be about 300 times as sweet as table sugar, and they have no added bulking agent, such as maltodextrin or dextrose (although the powdered form in packets does). Tablets are equivalent to half the sweetening power of the packets and come in a 100-tablet dispenser that can fit in purse or briefcase.

1 Equal tablet ≈ 1 teaspoon sugar in sweetening power

Acesulfame-K. Sunette or The Sweet One is said to be about 200 times sweeter than sugar, but it is not available in a liquid or tablet form. The powder contains the usual dextrose or maltodextrin additives for bulk. Its lack of availability without added sugar and its somewhat controversial status as a potential carcinogen make it less desirable than others. (Saccharin has been around for more than a century and has never been associated with cancer.)

Stevia. Stevia is the extract of an herb known by a variety of names, such as sweet herb. It comes in powder or liquid forms and is the only noncarbohydrate powdered sweetener that does not have added dextrose or maltodextrin. Extracts may vary in their sweetening power, depending on the maker.

Green stevia is less expensive than white, but to me the green has an unpleasant taste. If you can grow sweet herb, drying the leaves and using them in your tea, for example, can be a low-cost option.

Cyclamate. Cyclamate is said to be 30 times sweeter than sucrose. Available in other countries under brands such as

Sucaryl, cyclamate contains no calories. Sucaryl tablets and liquid, from Abbott Laboratories, contain cyclamate and saccharin.

1 Sucaryl tablet ≈ 1 teaspoon of sugar in sweetening power

Saccharin.   Saccharin is currently the least expensive of the artificial sweeteners. Saccharin is more than one hundred years old and so is available under a number of brands, in ½-grain and ¼-grain tablets and in inexpensive bottles of up to 1,000 tablets. You can also get bottles of saccharin liquid. Both ¼-grain tablets and the liquid form are available under the Sweet'n Low brand name.

1 Sweet'n Low tablet ≈ 1 teaspoon sugar in sweetening power
10 drops Sweet'n Low liquid ≈ 1 teaspoon sugar in sweetening
  power
2 tablespoons Sweet'n Low liquid ≈ 1 tablespoon sugar in
  sweetening power

Sucralose (Splenda).   Like other tabletop sweeteners except stevia, Splenda granular and packet products contain bulking ingredients — dextrose and/or maltodextrin, which are sugars. Splenda concentrate is available in the United States only to bulk manufacturers; the Splenda that sweetens Da Vinci syrups has no added dextrose or maltodextrin.

Da Vinci Gourmet Syrups

Da Vinci Gourmet makes a wide variety of sugared and sugar-free syrups. You can use the sugar-free variety (sweetened with Splenda) for everything from flavoring and sweetening yogurt to adding some pizzazz to your coffee, to adding flavor to your salad dressing or recipes. In my opinion this is the best product of its kind on the market. It's available from several Web distributors, including www.netrition. com and www.davincigourmet.com, and from Trotta's Pharmacy. Internet prices range from $7.49 to $8.95 for a 750 ml bottle. Da Vinci currently produces a wide variety of flavors, including banana, blueberry, caramel, cherry, choco-late, coconut, cookie dough, pancake, cola, vanilla, peanut butter, watermelon, and many more. I like to sometimes mix the toasted marshmallow syrup into my morning omelet. For a list of distributors, phone Da Vinci Gourmet, Ltd., at 800-640-6779. The product is certified kosher.

Flavor Extracts

There are numerous flavor extracts (vanilla, rum, orange, etc.) used in baking that you can use to make your food more interesting. They usually can be found in small brown bottles in the baking supply aisles of supermarkets. Read carbohydrate content from the label. Usually it's zero and therefore won't affect your blood sugar.

Mustard, Pepper, Salt, Spices, Herbs

Most commercial mustards are made without sugar and contain essentially no carbohydrate. This can readily be de-termined for a given brand by reading the label or by using the Clinistix/Diastix test. Pepper and salt have no effect upon blood sugar. Hypertensive individuals with proven salt sensitivity should, of course, avoid salt and highly salted foods (see page 439 in *Dr. Bernstein's Diabetes Solution,* 2003 edition).

Most herbs and spices have very low carbohydrate content and are used in such small amounts that the amount of ingested carbohydrate will be insignificant. Watch out, however, for certain combinations such as powdered cinnamon with sugar. Just read the labels.

Low-Carbohydrate Salad Dressings

Most salad dressings are loaded with sugars and other carbohydrates. The ideal dressing for someone who desires normal blood sugars would therefore be oil and vinegar, perhaps with added spices, mustard, and followed by grated cheese or even real or soy bacon bits. I like to add Da Vinci sugar-free raspberry syrup to mine.

There are now available some commercial salad dressings with only 1 gram carbohydrate per 2-tablespoon serving. This is low enough that such a product can be worked into our meal plans. Be careful with mayonnaise. Most brands are labeled "carbohydrate — 0 grams," but they may contain up to 0.4 grams per tablespoon. This is not a lot, but it adds up if you eat large amounts. Some imitation mayonnaise products have 5 grams of carbohydrate per 2-tablespoon serving.

Nuts

Although all nuts contain carbohydrate (as well as protein and fat), they usually raise blood sugar slowly and can in small amounts be worked into meal plans. As with most other foods, you will want to look up your favorite nuts in one of the books listed on page 52 in order to obtain their carbohydrate content. By way of example, 10 pistachio nuts (small, not jumbo) contain only 1 gram carbohydrate, while 10 cashew nuts contain 5 grams of carbohydrate. Although a few nuts may contain little carbohydrate, the catch is in the word "few." Very few of us can eat only a few nuts. In fact, I only have two patients who can count out a pre-planned number of nuts, eat them, and then stop. So unless you have unusual will power, beware. Also beware of peanut butter, another deceptive addiction. One tablespoon of natural, unsweetened peanut butter contains 3 grams of carbohydrate, which would raise my blood sugar modestly. Ten tablespoons would have a whopping effect.

Sugar-Free Jell-O Brand Gelatin

This is one of the few foods that in reasonable amounts will have almost no effect upon blood sugar — if you get the kind that is indeed sugar-free. Unfortunately, nowadays "sugar-free" powder actually contains some maltodextrin, which is a mixture of sugars and will raise your blood sugar. The ready-to-eat variety in plastic cups does not thus far contain maltodextrin — at least those I've found on my grocery's shelves. Check the labels. Truly sugar-free Jell-O or other truly sugar-free brands of gelatin are fine for snacks and desserts. A ½-cup serving contains no carbohydrate, no fat, and only 2 grams of protein. Limit yourself to no more than ½ cup twice daily and none at bedtime. My patients who eat sugar-free Jell-O at bedtime tend to experience an overnight blood sugar rise.

If the only "sugar-free" Jell-O you can find contains maltodextrin, try making your own by adding some liquid stevia and Da Vinci syrup to Knox unflavored gelatin as a tasty substitute.

Sugar-Free Jell-O Puddings

Available in chocolate, vanilla, pistachio, and butterscotch flavors, these make a nice dessert treat. These all contain a small amount of carbohydrate (about 6 grams per serving), which should be counted in your meal plan. Instead of mixing the powder with milk, which will raise the carbohydrate content, use water or water plus cream. Every 2 tablespoons of cream will add 1 gram of carbohydrate.

Chewing Gum

Gum chewing can be a good substitute for snacking and can be of value to people with gastroparesis because it stimulates salivation, releasing substances that facilitate stomach-emptying. The carbohydrate content of one stick of chewing gum varies from about 1 gram in a stick of sugar-free Trident or Orbit to about 7 grams per piece for some liquid-filled chewing gums. The 7-gram gum will rapidly raise my blood sugar. The carbohydrate content of a stick of chewing gum can usually be found on the package label. "Sugar-free" gums all contain small amounts of sugar. The primary ingredient of Trident "sugarless" gum is sorbitol, one of the stealth sugars from page 55 — actually, it's a corn-based sugar alcohol. Trident also includes mannitol and aspartame.

I frequently use a chewing gum called XlearDent. It contains about ¾ gram of the sugar xylitol per piece. Xylitol is an antimetabolite (metabolic poison) for bacteria and prevents tooth decay when chewed regularly. The gum may be obtained by phoning 877-599-5327, or on the Internet at www.xlear.com. Orbit also contains a small amount of xylitol and has more flavor that lasts longer than that of Trident or Xlear.

Truly Low Carbohydrate Desserts

This book includes 112 new low-carbohydrate recipes, created by chef and restaurateur Marcia Miele, who has learned the hard way how to "cook diabetic." Her son Dante, a type 1 diabetic, is a patient of mine. Her easy recipes for some low-carbohydrate desserts are truly delicious — for a kid who "can't have sweets," Marcia has had to be very creative.

Coffee, Tea, Seltzer, Mineral Water, Club Soda, Diet Sodas

None of these products should have significant effect upon blood sugar. Some of the popular low-carb diets say to eliminate coffee as much as possible. In theory, it should increase glucagon production and therefore raise blood sugar, but I have not seen it have an adverse effect on blood sugar when used in moderation. The coffee and tea may be sweetened with liquid or powdered stevia, or with *tablet* sweeteners such as saccharin, cyclamate, sucralose (Splenda tablets, if and when they arrive on the market), and aspartame (Equal tablets). Remember to avoid the use of more than 2 teaspoons of milk as a lightener. Try to use cream, which has much less carbohydrate, tastes better, and goes much further.

Read the labels of "diet" sodas, as a few brands contain sugar in the form of fruit juices. Many flavored mineral waters, bottled "diet" teas, and seltzers also contain added carbohydrate or sugar, as do many powdered beverages. Again, read the labels.

Frozen Diet Soda Pops

Many supermarkets and toy stores in the United States sell plastic molds for making your own ice pops. If these are filled with sugar-free sodas, you can create a tasty snack that has no effect upon blood sugar. Do not use the commercially made "sugar-free" or "diet" ice pops that are displayed in supermarket freezers. They contain fruit juices and other sources of carbohydrate.

Alcohol, in Limited Amounts

Ethyl alcohol (distilled spirits) has no direct effect upon blood sugar. Moderate amounts, however, can have a rapid effect upon the liver, preventing the conversion of dietary protein to glucose. If you are following a regimen that includes insulin or a pancreas-stimulating oral hypoglycemic agent, you're dependent upon conversion of protein to glucose in order to maintain blood sugar at safe levels. The effects of small amounts of alcohol (1½ ounces of spirits or 3 ounces of dry wine for a typical adult) are usually negligible.

Most beers (not stout or porter), in spite of their carbohydrate content, don't seem to affect blood sugar when only one can or bottle is consumed. If you like beer, try one, then check blood sugar hourly for the next 3 hours to see if the beer has caused an increase.

NUTRITION FACTS 101

Or, What's in What You Eat?

The single most widely recognizable graphic in the United States isn't a corporate logo like the Nike "swoosh" or a brand symbol like the cursive Coca-Cola name, it's a plain and unremarkable little box: the nutrition facts label. On virtually all packaged food and drink products, the graphic is ubiquitous in the United States.

The label can be a valuable source of information, but it can also be misleading or just dead wrong, depending on how the numbers were derived.

I rely heavily on food labels, and I encourage my patients — and you — to become an educated nutrition facts reader. Even though you can't always rely solely on nutrition labels, they are really the only source of information we have about many products. They can be inaccurate in a number of ways, starting with the numbers not adding up (a clue that the label may be unreliable), although sometimes the reason the numbers don't add up is due not to inaccuracy but to the way regulations require carbohydrate to be listed. It's mandatory that total carbohydrate be listed, as well as dietary fiber and sugar, but listing of sugar alcohols is optional. And since these numbers are all averages, there may be a margin of error; so if you add up all the smaller numbers under the total number, you may get a slightly different figure.

In addition, there are exceptions to the rules for the labels: small packages get an exemption and can use an abbreviated label; so can foods intended for children younger than four years and "medical foods, such as those used to address the nutritional needs of patients with certain diseases." Manufacturers can also "customize" their labels by using footnotes.

Of course there are also just plain mistakes and even outright misrepresentations. I've seen strawberry preserves that are labeled as zero carbohydrate when it is obvious, from the berries in the jar, that there is plenty of carbohydrate. Mistakes can also happen with respect to foods that originate in the European Union and have had labels (with differing regulatory requirements) "translated" into American nutrition facts labels. And then there are good old typos — numbers that are incorrect or have misplaced decimal points.

The good news is that FDA spot checks have supposedly shown that overall, better than 90 percent of the time, the labels are accurate.

THE NUTRITION LABELING and Education Act of 1990 established standards for the information included on these labels.* Interestingly, the labels were in part a government response to the low-fat craze. The two most prominent numbers are for carbohydrate and fat, which have overall totals, but also have a breakdown — fiber and sugars, and saturated and unsaturated fats.

Manufacturers are required to measure several categories: protein, fat, carbohydrate, particular nutrients (select vitamins, as well as iron and calcium), and calories. The tricky thing about these labels is that there are different ways the information can be assembled. The maker can

---

*A very comprehensive explanation of nutrition facts labeling can be found on the FDA's Web site. Look on www.fda.gov and search for information on nutrition facts labeling.

send the product off to the lab for an actual (averaged) measurement of protein, fat, and carbohydrate (see below), or it can estimate based on the ingredients in the recipe (as we do in creating meal plans).

Neither method is absolutely precise, but since every person can react to foods differently, and exact measurements would likely be quite expensive, absolutely precise measurements aren't necessary.

There are standards for lab analyses of the different categories of nutrients in foods. There may be more than one approved method, and one method may be more precise than another. Each, however, has its limitations. One manufacturer of chicken soup, for example, may analyze the product in a lab. Another may use the recipe. The latter could, for example, use a proprietary database of nutrition information, or it could use a public resource like the U.S. Department of Agriculture's National Nutrient Database. Since there is no single bible of nutritional information from which the data are derived, there will be variations depending on the source.

Say you're shopping for breakfast sausage. You look at three different products. All have exactly the same ingredients except for salt and their special blend of spices. Two use their own labs to test their products and the other uses the recipe method. The likelihood of discrepancy is high.

That doesn't necessarily mean, however, that the differences will be enormous, or even noticeable. Chances are good that the nutrition analyses are going to be very similar. If they aren't — if the labels list significantly different amounts of protein, carbohydrate, or fat — a simple mistake, rather than the methodology, is likely to be the cause.

How Do They Do It?

In the lab, protein is estimated based on a test of nitrogen. As you may know, protein is made up of amino acids. Each amino acid contains a nitrogen atom, so a lab can accurately estimate protein content by the amount of nitrogen in the food. Fat content is estimated based on the weight of the fatty acids (lipids) present in the product. For every three fatty acids, the lab adds the weight of a glycerol molecule. This provides a pretty accurate picture of triglyceride (fat) content, since three fatty acid molecules plus one glycerol molecule equals one triglyceride molecule.

Fat must be further broken down into saturated and unsaturated, and new requirements require listing trans fat (as in hydrogenated vegetable oil, for example). Carbohydrate is measured last, and it's done by elimination — overall weight of the food minus protein, fat, water, and ash equals carbohydrate. Carbohydrate must also be broken down into fiber and sugar. Measuring the amount and type of carbohydrate in food is a complicated business and requires sophisticated chemistry for some carbohydrate, while for others, such as pure starch or sugar, reasonably simple enzymatic treatment can be used.

In addition, some nutrition information is just not provided on the labels. The list below shows the "facts" that food manufacturers are allowed to include on the nutrition label. The items in boldface are mandatory, the others are optional.

- **total calories**
- **calories from fat**
- calories from saturated fat
- **total fat**
- **saturated fat**

- **trans fat**
- polyunsaturated fat
- monounsaturated fat
- **cholesterol**
- **sodium**
- potassium
- **total carbohydrate**
- **dietary fiber**
- soluble fiber
- insoluble fiber
- **sugars**
- sugar alcohol (for example, the sugar substitutes xylitol, mannitol, and sorbitol)
- other carbohydrate (the difference between total carbohydrate and the sum of dietary fiber, sugars, and sugar alcohol if declared)
- **protein**
- **vitamin A**
- percent of vitamin A present as beta-carotene
- **vitamin C**
- **calcium**
- **iron**
- other essential vitamins and minerals

According to the FDA explanation of the regulations:

If a claim is made about any of the optional components, or if a food is fortified or enriched with any of them, nutrition information for these components becomes mandatory.

These mandatory and voluntary components are *the only ones allowed* [emphasis added] on the Nutrition Facts panel.* The listing of single amino acids, maltodextrin, calories from polyunsaturated fat, and calories from carbohydrates, for example, may not appear as part of the Nutrition Facts on the label.

The required nutrients were selected because they address today's health concerns. The order in which they must appear reflects the priority of current dietary recommendations.†

It's interesting to note that maltodextrin (a mixture of sugars derived from corn) "may not appear" on the nutrition facts label (it can and does appear on the ingredients list). It's also worth noting the reference to "current dietary recommendations." This has permitted occasional regulatory amendments (trans fats were added in 2003, for example), and it would not be surprising to see labeling requirements amended again as "current dietary recommendations" and "today's health concerns" continue to evolve.

Read Labels

As you now know, virtually all packaged foods bear labels that reveal something about the contents; you also know that the FDA requires the labels of packaged foods to list the amount of carbohydrate, protein, fat, and fiber in a serving. Be sure, however, to note the size of the "serving." For some foods, the serving size is so small that you wouldn't want to be bothered eating it. The FDA explains that the

---

*But that doesn't mean they can't use footnotes.
†"The Food Label." FDA Backgrounder, May 1999. See the full text at www.cfsan.fda.gov/~dms/fdnewlab.html.

nutrition labeling law "defines serving size as the amount of food customarily eaten at one time. The serving sizes that appear on food labels are based on FDA-established lists of 'Reference Amounts Customarily Consumed Per Eating Occasion.'" You might think, for example, that a single bottle of soda would be considered one serving. Look again. If it's an 8- or even 12-ounce bottle, you'd be right. But the regulations allow manufacturers some wiggle room, and some 20-ounce bottles list the contents as three servings. In my opinion, this latitude can be used to mislead without being legally dishonest.

Beware of labels that say "lite," "light," "sugar-free," "dietetic," "diet," "reduced-calorie," "low calorie," "low fat," "fat-free," and even "low carbohydrate." Although the Nutrition Labeling and Education Act establishes standards for some of these categories, and likely will soon adopt a standard for "low carbohydrate," that standard, like the rest, will likely be essentially meaningless for those who are diabetic, overweight, or obese and in need of particularly clear information about what's in what they eat. These tags can be used as smoke and mirrors to distract you from the hard facts.

There are several things to keep in mind:

- Counts of calories are only going to tell you so much, as discussed on page 41.
- "Low fat" tells you nothing about carbohydrate content.
- "Fat-free" products — desserts and similar products — frequently contain considerable fast-acting carbohydrate to make up for the loss of flavor from the absent fat.

- Even if you're losing weight, carbohydrate intake will impede your efforts much more than fat will. Two recent studies showed that when dietary carbohydrate is very low, dietary fat is metabolized, not stored. (On occasion I see slim patients whose desire is to gain weight. I've found that it's impossible to put weight on those who are following a low-carbohydrate diet even by giving them *900 extra calories* a day in the form of 4 ounces of olive oil.)

- Use common sense about nutrition facts claims. The common way to estimate the carbohydrate content of a particular food is to read the amount stated on the label. "Sugar-free," remember, does not mean carbohydrate-free. As mentioned above, I know of a brand of strawberry preserves whose label claims, "Carbohydrate — 0," and yet anyone can see the strawberries in the jar. Strawberries are mostly carbohydrate, so unless those are artificially flavored hunks of tenderloin made to look like strawberries (unlikely), common sense would tell you that the label is flat-out wrong. Deceptive labeling does occur and in my experience is fairly prevalent in the "diet" food industry.

Use Food Value Manuals

On page 52, I listed a few books that show the approximate carbohydrate and protein contents of various foods. These manuals are recommended but not essential tools for creating your meal plan. The meal plan guidelines in the next chapter, the recipes that follow, and the advice in the preceding pages are all you really need to get started. Those manuals are great when you're creating your own recipes and want to get the carbohydrate and protein numbers.

My favorite is *The NutriBase Complete Book of Food Counts,* because it contains information on the most brands and is easy to use.

Food Values of Portions Commonly Used has been the dietitian's bible for more than fifty years and is updated every few years. Be sure to use the index at the back to locate the foods of interest. Note that on every page in the main section, carbohydrate and fat content are listed in the same column. The carbohydrate content of a food always appears below the fat content. Do not get the two confused. **Be sure to note the portion size in any books you use.**

If you watch cooking shows, you've probably seen chefs who keep a computer handy while they're cooking. If you're electronically inclined, you can use the USDA's nutrient database, which you can find on the Web by searching on the key words "USDA nutrient database." The USDA now offers free software for the National Nutrient Database for Windows OS computers and for Palm OS personal digital assistants (PDAs) on both the Windows and Macintosh platforms. You can download the software at www.nal. usda.gov/fnic/foodcomp/srch/search.htm. This has the potential to be a great tool for those who travel and carry PDAs.

VITAMIN AND MINERAL SUPPLEMENTS

It is common practice to prescribe supplementary vitamins and minerals for diabetics. This is primarily because most diabetics have chronically high blood sugars and therefore urinate a lot. Excessive urination causes a loss of water-soluble vitamins and minerals. If you can keep your blood sugars low enough to avoid spilling glucose into the urine (you can test it with Clinistix or Diastix), and if you eat a variety of vegetables, and red meat at least once or twice a week, you should not require supplements. Note, however, that major dietary sources of B-complex vitamins (folic acid is one of these) include "fortified" or supplemented breads and grains in the United States. If you're following a low-carbohydrate diet and therefore exclude these from your meal plan, you should eat some bean sprouts, spinach, broccoli, brussels sprouts, or cauliflower each day. If you do not like vegetables, you might take a B-complex capsule or a multivitamin/mineral capsule each day.

Supplemental vitamins and minerals should not ordinarily be used in excess of the FDA's recommended daily requirements. Large doses can inhibit the body's synthesis of some vitamins and intestinal absorption of certain minerals. Large doses are also potentially toxic. Doses of vitamin C in excess of 500 mg daily may interfere with blood sugar readings (causing them to appear erroneously low). Large doses of vitamin C can actually raise blood sugar, cause kidney stones, and even impair nerve function (as can doses of vitamin B-6 in excess of 200 mg daily, so beware of B-complex capsules). Vitamin E has been shown to reduce one of the destructive effects of high blood sugars (glycosylation of the body's proteins),* with increased amounts providing increased benefit up to 1,200 IU (international units) per day.

---

*Glycosylation of protein — the bonding of glucose to protein — is essentially what you see in bread crust. Inside the bread loaf the proteins are supple, but the proteins in the crust have bonded with sugars and lost any resilience. Bad news when it happens inside your body.

It has recently been shown to lower insulin resistance. I therefore recommend 400–1,200 IU per day to a number of my patients. Be sure to use the forms of vitamin E known as gamma tocopherol or mixed tocopherols, not the common alpha tocopherol, which can inhibit the absorption of essential gamma tocopherol from foods. Vitamin E can reduce the ability of blood to clot and must therefore be restricted in some people. Consult your physician before using it.

The insulin-sensitizing agent metformin can cause systemic reduction of vitamin B-12. This can be corrected with calcium supplements or more calcium in your diet (cream or cheese, for example).

CHANGES IN BOWEL MOVEMENTS

A new diet often brings about changes in frequency and consistency of bowel movements. This is perfectly natural and should not cause concern unless you experience discomfort. Increasing the fiber content of meals, as with salads, bran crackers, and soybean products, can cause softer and more frequent stools. More dietary protein can cause less frequent and harder stools. Calcium supplements can cause hard stools and constipation, but this is usually offset if they contain magnesium. Normal frequency of bowel movements can range from 3 times per day to 3 times per week. If you notice any changes in your bowel habits more or less than these frequencies, discuss them with your physician.

HOW DO PEOPLE REACT
TO THE NEW DIET?

Most of my patients initially feel somewhat deprived, but they are also grateful to feel more alert and healthier — sometimes more so than they have in years. I fall into this category myself. My mouth waters whenever I pass a bakery shop and sniff the aroma of fresh bread, but I am also grateful simply to be alive and sniffing.

5

Customizing the Diet

If you found yourself thinking as you went through the No-No foods section in Chapter 3 that all of this information goes against conventional thinking — you're right. For years, "heart-attack food" was synonymous with red meat, eggs, and butter. The evidence is in. That is utterly and completely wrong.

Fast-acting, concentrated carbohydrate is the ultimate heart-attack food, particularly for those with a sedentary lifestyle.

It used to be that my patients faced an uphill battle with their friends and family, who were convinced that my advice was wrong, or wanted them to try more "fun" foods. The low-carbohydrate craze has changed that somewhat, but you may still face well-meaning but uninformed friends and family who want you to eat less "bad fat" and more "complex" carbohydrates.

You can patiently express appreciation for their affection and care but ignore their advice. When they see you looking healthier, slimmer, fitter, and more energetic than you have in years, they might just ask to borrow this book.

It's a good idea, before you start, to get a baseline measure of your cardiac risk and renal (kidney) profile. When you get a follow-up measure six months later, you'll demonstrate conclusively that our diet has lowered both classes of risk factors. It doesn't matter whether you're diabetic, overweight, or obese. There is, however, one caveat. Autoimmune disorders such as diabetes are usually found in clusters. So, for example, it is not unusual for diabetics to develop a low thyroid state (hypothyroidism) either before or after they develop diabetes. This can occur at any age and will absolutely increase several cardiac risk factors, such as LDL, homocysteine, and lipoprotein(a). Fortunately, thyroid supplementation can reverse this condition. (Most physicians, however, perform the wrong thyroid function test. See page 435 of *Diabetes Solution*, 2003 edition.)

GENERAL PRINCIPLES FOR TAILORING YOUR MEAL PLAN

If you use blood sugar–lowering medications such as insulin or oral agents, the first rule of meal planning is: Don't change your diet unless your physician first reviews the new meal plan and reduces your medications accordingly. Most diabetics who begin our low-carbohydrate diet show an immediate and dramatic drop in blood sugar levels after meals, as compared to blood sugars on their prior, high-carbohydrate diets. *If at the same time your medications are not appropriately reduced, your blood sugars can drop to dangerously low levels.*

Your meal plan should be geared toward blood sugar control — and weight loss if you're overweight — and also toward keeping you content with what you eat. So with those things in mind, one of the first things I do when I "train" my patients is "negotiate" a meal plan with them.

I say "negotiate" because I have never seen a one-size-fits-all diet work. One person may find the idea of sardines for breakfast delightful, another may find it disgusting. To work up an individualized plan, we start by making a list of what you eat and when, including snacks, on a typical day.*

If you're a diabetic, I would also ask you to provide me with data sheets showing your blood sugar profiles, meals, and any blood sugar–lowering medications you'd taken during the previous week or two. These sheets should include any physical exercise you may have performed. My patients and I use GLUCOGRAF II data sheets (see page 111) for this purpose. (You'll find their use detailed in Chapter 5 of *Diabetes Solution*.)† We would also take into account your height, weight, and age.

This information would give me an idea of what you like to eat and what effect particular doses of blood sugar–lowering medications have on your blood sugars.

Other important factors I take into account:

- If you have delayed stomach-emptying
- If you're taking medications for other ailments that might affect your blood sugar

In negotiating the meal plan, I'd try wherever possible to incorporate foods you like. There are no prescribed

---

*I don't recommend snacks for diabetics who use insulin to correct elevated blood sugars before meals.
†Pads of blank data sheets covering an entire year are available through Trotta's Pharmacy, www.trottaspharmacy.com, phone 877-987-6882.

meals. There is only one absolutely hard and fast rule: Avoid fast-acting, concentrated carbohydrate.

If you've tried dieting to lose weight or to get your diabetes under control, you may have found that simply cutting back on calories according to preprinted tables or fixed calculations can be frustrating and can even have the opposite effect.

If your "diet" calls for a supper that doesn't satisfy you, it's almost a given that later on you'll find yourself compelled to have a snack. If you're like most people, your snack will be snack food, a bowl of cereal, a banana, a bowl of ice cream — in other words, something loaded with fast-acting carbohydrate. The result? You end up with high blood sugars and more calories than you would have consumed if you'd started with a sensible meal.

My aim is to help you avoid this. It's best to start with a plan that allows you to get up from the table feeling comfortable but not stuffed. Studies have shown that fat and protein both leave you considerably more satisfied than fast-acting carbohydrate.

Since all of my diabetic patients bring me glucose profiles, over the years it has not been very difficult to develop guidelines for carbohydrate consumption that make blood sugar control relatively easy without causing too great a feeling of deprivation, even for those trying to lose weight.

6-12-12

My basic approach in helping someone put together a meal plan is that I first set carbohydrate amounts for each meal.

The general parameters work like this. I recommend

GlucograF II DATA SHEET

© 2000 Richard K. Bernstein, M.D., Mamaroneck, NY 10543

Name:

DOCTOR'S PHONE	USUAL DOSES OF INSULIN OR ORAL AGENT
DOCTOR'S FAX	Upon Arising ___
	Min. pre / post bkfst. ___
	Min. pre / post lunch ___
TARGET	Min. pre / post dinner ___
BG	Min. pre / post snacks ___
	At Bedtime

1 Unit H will Lower Blood Sugar ___ mg/dl

MISCELLANEOUS

BG EFFECTS OF SWEETS (mg/dl)

1 gm CHO →

EXERCISE ADJUSTMENTS

ABBREVIATIONS
B- Breakfast
Ex- Exercise
H- Humalog Insulin
IM- Intramuscular
L- Lente Insulin
LAN- Lantus Insulin
LU- Lunch
R- Regular Insulin
S- Supper
SN- Snack
UL- Ultralente Insulin

DATE WEEK BEGINS / /	SUNDAY			MONDAY			TUESDAY			WEDNESDAY			THURSDAY			FRIDAY			SATURDAY		
	TIME	BLOOD SUGAR	MEDICATION EXERCISE, FOOD, etc.	TIME	BLOOD SUGAR	MEDICATION EXERCISE, FOOD, etc.	TIME	BLOOD SUGAR	MEDICATION EXERCISE, FOOD, etc.	TIME	BLOOD SUGAR	MEDICATION EXERCISE, FOOD, etc.	TIME	BLOOD SUGAR	MEDICATION EXERCISE, FOOD, etc.	TIME	BLOOD SUGAR	MEDICATION EXERCISE, FOOD, etc.	TIME	BLOOD SUGAR	MEDICATION EXERCISE, FOOD, etc.
1 AM THRU 6 AM																					
6 AM THRU 9 AM																					
9 AM THRU 12 NOON																					
12 NOON THRU 3 PM																					
3 PM THRU 6 PM																					
6 PM THRU 9 PM																					
9 PM THRU 1 AM																					

restricting their carbohydrate to about 6 grams of slow-acting carbohydrate at breakfast, 12 grams at lunch, and 12 grams at supper. Very few people would be willing to eat less. (These guidelines also apply to children.) The limitation of only 6 at breakfast is because of the Dawn Phenomenon (page 33), but it really isn't hard to stick to.

A recent study of overweight children found that when three groups were fed three different breakfasts — a high-carbohydrate breakfast; a so-called complex-carbohydrate breakfast; and a high-fat, low-carb breakfast — those in the last group had the highest sense of satisfaction for the longest period of time after their meal. Those in the first two groups were more prone to feeling the "need" to snack.

When we've established parameters for carbohydrate, then we talk about how many ounces of protein, in addition to the carbohydrate, we should add to make you feel satisfied. (If you came into my office, I'd show you plastic samples of protein foods of various sizes, to give you an idea of what various amounts actually look like.)

There is no such thing as an essential carbohydrate for normal development, despite what the popular press might have you believe about the health benefits of "complex" carbohydrate. There most certainly are proteins we must have (essential amino acids) and fats (essential fatty acids). We include carbohydrates in the meal plan not just because you might not enjoy the meals without them, but because in addition to the vitamins and minerals present in vegetables there are many other nonvitamin chemicals — phytochemicals — that have only recently become understood. These are crucial to good nutrition and cannot be obtained through conventional vitamin supplements. Some phytochemicals, such as beta carotene, are highly beneficial when consumed in plant form but may actually be harmful if taken in supplements. There are still many things that remain unclear about phytochemicals. In terms of beneficial phytochemicals, whole-plant and leaf varieties of vegetables are particularly good sources. Folic acid — as noted previously, so named because it is derived from foliage — is essential to all manner of development, but strictly speaking it is considered neither vitamin nor mineral.

Ideally, your blood sugar should be the same after eating as it was before. If blood sugar increases after a meal, even if it eventually drops to your target value, either the meal content should be changed or blood sugar–lowering medications should be used before you eat.

Slow-Acting Carbohydrate

As I have mentioned before, the distinction often made between "complex" and "simple" carbohydrates is essentially meaningless, if not foolish. There are fast-acting carbohydrates — starches and sugars that break down rapidly and have a consequent rapid effect on blood sugars — and there are slow-acting carbohydrates. Generally, slow-acting carbohydrate comes from whole-plant vegetables (and others listed on page 77). They are predominantly indigestible fiber accompanied by some small amount of digestible carbohydrate and vitamins, minerals, and other compounds, but have relatively little effect on blood sugars.

The foods in the following list are slow-acting carbohydrate foods. These can constitute the building blocks of the carbohydrate portion of each meal. Of course you needn't limit your foods to these — many other such building blocks can be selected, depending on your personal preferences.

Read labels on packaged foods, consult nutrition tables for carbohydrate values of foods you like, check your blood sugars, and find out which foods work for you.

Equivalent to approximately 6 grams of carbohydrate per serving

- 6 Worthington Stripples or Morningstar Farms Breakfast Strips (meatless soy bacon) (also contains 1 ounce protein)
- 3 Morningstar Farms Breakfast Links (meatless soy sausage) (also contains 2 ounces protein)
- 1½ Bran-a-Crisp crackers
- 2 GG crispbreads
- 1 Wasa Fiber Rye cracker
- 4½ ounces Erivan, Brown Cow Farm, or Stonyfield Farm whole-milk unflavored yogurt (8 ounces contains 11 grams carbohydrate and 2 ounces protein)
- 1 cup mixed salad with oil-and-vinegar (not balsamic) dressing
- ⅔ cup cooked slow-acting carbohydrate vegetable — zucchini, mushrooms, eggplant, etc. (see The List on page 77)
- 1 serving Jell-O sugar-free pudding made with water or water and 1 tablespoon cream
- ½ small avocado (3 ounces)

Equivalent to approximately 12 grams of carbohydrate per serving

- 1 cup mixed salad with oil-and-vinegar (not balsamic) dressing, plus ⅔ cup cooked green vegetable (from page 77)

- 1 cup mixed salad prepared with 4 tablespoons packaged dressing (if each tablespoon contains 1.5 grams of carbohydrate)
- 8 ounces Erivan, Brown Cow Farm, or Stonyfield Farm whole-milk unflavored yogurt (contains 11 grams of carbohydrate plus 2 ounces protein)

These lists slightly exaggerate the carbohydrate content of salad and cooked vegetables, but because of their bulk and the Chinese Restaurant Effect, the net effect upon blood sugar is approximately equivalent to the amounts of carbohydrate shown. To this slow-acting carbohydrate, we'd add an amount of protein that, in your initial opinion, would allow you to leave the table feeling comfortable but not stuffed.

Protein

As with carbohydrate, it is necessary to keep the size of the protein portion at a particular meal constant from one day to the next, so if you eat 6 ounces at lunch one day, you should have 6 ounces at lunch the next. This is especially important if you're taking blood sugar–lowering medications. As noted earlier, there are about 6 grams of real protein in an ounce of a protein food. So when you are using tables of food values in creating your own Diabetes Diet meal plans, remember to divide *grams* of protein by 6 to get the equivalent *ounces* of protein food. To estimate by eye, a cooked portion the size of a deck of playing cards or a small can of tuna fish weighs about 3 ounces (red meats weigh about 3.7 ounces because of their greater density).

Protein foods with virtually no carbohydrate

- Beef, lamb, veal
- Chicken, turkey, duck
- Most cold cuts (bologna, salami, etc.)
- Fish and shellfish (fresh or canned)
- Most frankfurters
- Pork (ham, chops, bacon, etc.)
- Most sausages

Protein foods with a small amount of carbohydrate (0.6–1 gram carbohydrate per ounce of protein)

- Eggs (one egg is equivalent to 1 ounce protein plus 0.6 gram carbohydrate); include the carbohydrate content when calculating the carbohydrate portion of a meal
- Cheeses (other than cottage cheese); the 1 gram of carbohydrate per ounce found in most cheeses should be included when computing the carbohydrate portion of a meal

Soy products (up to 6 grams carbohydrate per ounce of protein — check nutrition label on package)

- Veggie burgers
- Tofu
- Meatless bacon
- Meatless sausage
- Other soy substitutes (for fish, chicken, and so on)

If you have a rare disorder called familial dyslipidemia, where dietary fat actually can increase LDL, restrictions on certain types of dietary fats may be appropriate.

THE TIMING OF MEALS AND SNACKS

Meals need not follow a rigidly fixed time schedule, provided that, in most cases, you do not begin eating within
4 hours of the end of the prior meal. It takes 4–5 hours for
the effect of a meal on blood sugar to run its course. When
you have overlapping blood sugar effects, it is more difficult
to control blood sugar. If you eat your breakfast meal at
seven in the morning but then an hour later eat a high-carbohydrate snack, the bottom line is that you will prolong the
need for high levels of insulin to "cover" the carbohydrate.
If your breakfast is a low-carbohydrate meal but then you
snack on a bagel or bun an hour or two later, you will
negate whatever virtue the low-carbohydrate meal had. The
added insulin needed to cover the blood sugar spike from
the snack will help pack away the fat you ate, when otherwise it would have been metabolized. (When a patient is a
snacker, he's obese and his blood sugars are uncontrollable.)

If you do not take insulin, you need not be restricted to
only three daily meals if you prefer four or more similar
meals on a regular basis. The timing, again, should ideally
be at least 4 hours after the end of the prior meal or snack.
For most type 2 diabetics, it may be easier to control blood
sugar, with or without medication, after eating several smaller
meals than after eating only one or two large meals. Those
diabetics who use rapid-acting injected insulin to lower
blood sugar before meals must wait at least 5 hours between insulin injections and therefore between meals.

Remember that there are no diabetes-related restrictions
on coffee and tea, either plain or with cream (not milk) and/
or liquid or tablet (not powdered, except for stevia) sweeteners.

Now, let's put the guidelines to work in some practical examples.

CREATING YOUR OWN MEAL PLANS

Most people are creatures of habit and tend to eat the same thing every day for breakfast or lunch. I've had patients who have eaten the same toasted bialy for twenty years for breakfast, the same ham and cheese sandwich for lunch. In my experience, most of the variation people have in their diet comes at dinner. But let's start with breakfast. In my experience, bacon-and-egg people tend to eat bacon and eggs almost every day, maybe varying somewhat on weekends. Cereal people tend to eat cereal every day, even if they happen to change brands or flavors. Same with bagel people.

One of the problems with most of the popular low-carb diets on the market these days is that they introduce "habits" you would never take up on your own and then, just as you get used to them, move on to a new phase with different foods. So during phase one you might have vegetable juice, a protein food like liquid egg substitute or Canadian bacon, and coffee or tea. But most of the popular diets change to phase two after weight loss has been attained. This usually involves reverting to an approximation of old habits, such as those in the first paragraph. This is certainly not a way to keep blood sugars normal or to prevent recurrence of carbohydrate craving.

Right off the top, you know that I wouldn't recommend skim milk or vegetable juice, and I would recommend liquid egg substitute only if that was something you liked.

So, what *do* you like to eat?

There was a time in the American consciousness when fixing a meal was as simple as putting together a serving of protein, one of starch, and one of vegetables, with perhaps a side of salad and a small dessert. That standard menu — a piece of meat next to mashed potatoes, green beans, and tossed salad — made meal planning a simple proposition.

What I'm advocating is really as easy to conceive as the old meat, potatoes, vegetable, salad picture — just leave out the potato.

While the columns of numbers in the typical meal plans that follow may seem a little intimidating at first, in truth, once you become accustomed to the guidelines, putting together a meal — without having to consult a cookbook for every meal — becomes a simple process.

Breakfast

I recommend eating breakfast every day, especially if you're overweight. In my experience, most obese people have a history of either skipping or eating very little breakfast. They get hungry later in the day and overeat. That's a habit you should try to change right away. For most of us, any meal can be skipped, but if you're using blood sugar–lowering medication, you have to take that into account.

A typical breakfast on our meal plan would include up to 6 grams carbohydrate and an amount of protein to be determined by you. The amount of protein you "negotiate" per meal will remain constant from day to day. The best place to start is with what you currently eat, as long as it's not on the No-No list (see pages 58–61).

Suppose that, like many of my new patients, you've been eating a bagel loaded with cream cheese and 2 cups of coffee with skim milk and Sweet'n Low powdered sweetener for breakfast (totaling about 40 grams of rapid-acting carbohydrates). As we negotiate, I might propose that you substitute other sweeteners for the Sweet'n Low and 1 ounce WestSoy soymilk (0.5 gram carbohydrate) or cream (1 gram carbohydrate) for the skim milk in each cup of coffee.

Instead of a bagel I'd suggest you try one Bran-a-Crisp cracker (4 grams carbohydrate) with 1 ounce of cream cheese (1 gram carbohydrate plus 1 ounce protein). This adds up to about 6 grams of carbohydrate. Finally, I'd suggest that you add a protein food to your meal to make up for the calories and "filling power" that disappeared with the bagel. This could take almost any form, from lox to ham to a hotdog — or two. (See the lists on page 116.)

If you're a bacon-and-egg person but have been eating a side order of two slices of toast with jelly, I'd ask what it would take to make you feel satisfied after giving up the toast and jelly. You might add one Bran-a-Crisp cracker or a cheese puff (page 172) instead.

Or you might want to make the Quick Breakfast Omelet (page 164) with three eggs instead of two, which would give you about 4 grams of carbohydrate (to which you could add some scallions or chives or herbs), instead of eating one of the carbohydrate foods mentioned above.

If you're unnecessarily afraid of the cholesterol in egg yolks, you might use organic eggs or egg whites. If you find egg whites bland, you could add spices, or soy or Tabasco sauce, or some mushrooms or a small amount of onion or cheese, or chili powder, or even cinnamon with stevia, to enhance the taste. One of my current personal favorites for flavoring is a "chili sauce" made from Better Than Bouillon chili base, which is in the Low-Carb Chili recipe on page 218, and which you can get in most supermarkets. This packs a nice chili punch with very little carbohydrate (according to the label, 1 gram of carbohydrate per 2 teaspoons) and works quite well on eggs or other foods, depending on your tastes. (I like to make chili burgers with it — which you could certainly have for breakfast or any other meal.)

Lunch

Follow the same guidelines for lunch as for breakfast, with the exception that the carbohydrate content may be doubled, up to 12 grams.

Say, for example, that you and your friends go to lunch every day at the "greasy spoon" around the corner from work and are served only sandwiches. You might try discarding the slices of bread and eating the filling — meat, turkey, cheese, or other protein food — with a knife and fork. (If you choose cheese, remember to count 1 gram carbohydrate per ounce.) You could also order a hamburger without the bun. And instead of ketchup, you could use mustard, soy sauce, or other carbohydrate-free condiments. You then might add 1⅓ cups cooked vegetable from The List, page 77 (12 grams carbohydrate), or 2 cups of salad with vinegar-and-oil dressing (12 grams of carbohydrate) to round out your meal.

If you want to create a lunch menu from scratch, use your food value books to look up foods that interest you. If you like sandwiches, try the Cheese Puff Sandwich recipe on page 172.

The following building blocks may be helpful in giving you a start.

For the protein portion, one of the following

- A small can of tuna fish contains 3¼ ounces by weight in the United States. If you're packing your lunch, this can be quite convenient if you like tuna. The next larger size can contains 6 ounces. The tastiest canned tuna I've tried is made by Progresso, packed in olive oil.
- 4 standard slices of packaged pasteurized process American cheese (process cheddar in the U.K.) weigh about 3 ounces. This will contain 3 ounces of protein and 3 grams of carbohydrate.

For about 12 grams carbohydrate, one of the following

- 1⅓ cups cooked vegetables (from page 77).
- 2 cups mixed green salad, with 1 slice of tomato and vinegar-and-oil dressing. Sprinkling bacon bits or grated cheese will have negligible additional blood sugar effect.
- 1½ cups salad, as above, but with 3 tablespoons of commercial salad dressing (other than simple vinegar-and-oil) containing 1 gram of carbohydrate per tablespoon. Check the label.

You might decide that 2 cups of salad with vinegar-and-oil dressing is fine for the carbohydrate portion of your lunch. You then should decide how much protein must be added to keep you satisfied. One person might be happy with a 3¼-ounce can of tuna fish, but another might require 2 large chicken drumsticks or a packet of lunch meat weighing 6 ounces. For dessert, you might want some cheese (in the European tradition) or perhaps some sugar-free Jell-O gelatin (if it contains no maltodextrin) covered with 2 tablespoons of heavy cream. You might consider some of the desserts described in Part Two. The possible combinations are endless; just use your food value books or read labels for estimating protein and carbohydrate. Some people, after having routinely eaten the same thing for years, discover that their new meal plan opens up culinary possibilities they never knew existed.

Supper

Supper should follow essentially the same approach as lunch. There is, however, one significant difference that will only apply to those who are affected by delayed stomach-emptying (gastroparesis) and take insulin. As we've discussed briefly, this condition can cause unpredictable shifts in blood sugar levels because food doesn't always pass into the intestines at the same rate from meal to meal, which means that you can end up with unpredictably high or low blood sugars while you are sleeping and unable to monitor and correct them. A more complete analysis of this problem appears in Chapter 22 of *Dr. Bernstein's Diabetes Solution*.

If you like cooked vegetables (from The List) for supper, remember that most can be interchanged with salads as near equivalents — ⅔ cup of cooked vegetable and 1 cup of salad each have the blood sugar effect of about 6 grams carbohydrate.

If you like wine with dinner, choose a very dry variety and limit yourself to one 3-ounce glass. One beer may actually turn out to have no effect upon your blood sugar. Still, don't drink more than one.

Snacks

For many people with diabetes, snacks should be neither mandatory nor forbidden. They do, however, pose a problem for people who take fast-acting insulin before meals. Snacks should be a convenience, to relieve hunger if meals are delayed or spaced too far apart for comfort. If your diabetes is severe enough to warrant the use of rapid-acting blood sugar–lowering medication before meals, such medication may also be necessary before snacks.

The carbohydrate limit of 6 grams during the first few hours after arising and 12 grams of carbohydrate thereafter that applies to meals also applies to snacks. Be sure that your prior meal has been fully digested before your snack starts (this usually means waiting 4–5 hours). This is so that the effects upon blood sugar will not add to one another.

You needn't worry, however, if the snack is so sparse (say, a bit of toasted nori) as to have negligible effects on blood sugar. Sugar-free Jell-O gelatin (without maltodextrin) can be consumed pretty much whenever you like, provided you don't stuff yourself and provoke the Chinese Restaurant Effect. As a rule, snacks limited to small amounts of protein will have less effect upon blood sugar than those containing carbohydrate. Thus 2–3 ounces of cheese or cold cuts might be reasonable snacks for some people.

SOME TYPICAL MEAL PLANS

The following are typical meal plans covering 3 days. Note that the protein portions that this hypothetical person negotiated are 5 ounces for breakfast, 8 ounces for lunch, and 8 ounces for dinner. She is also following the 6-12-12 guidelines for carbohydrate.

Day One

Breakfast	Carbohydrate (*grams*)	Protein (*ounces*)
Scrambled Eggs with Zucchini and Cheddar (page 167)	6.3	3.3
2 ounces ham	–	2.0
TOTAL	6.3	5.3

Lunch

	Carbohydrate (*grams*)	Protein (*ounces*)
Lobster Salad (page 178)	10.9	6.3
1 Peanut Butter Cookie (page 274)	2.5	0.6
TOTAL	13.4	6.9

Supper

	Carbohydrate (*grams*)	Protein (*ounces*)
Salad with Artichokes, Hearts of Palm, Bacon, and Blue Cheese (page 181)	8.7	3.85
Filet au Poivre (page 221)	3.6	4.32
TOTAL	12.3	8.17

Day Two

Breakfast	Carbohydrate (*grams*)	Protein (*ounces*)
Bran cracker "cereal" made by crumbling 2 GG crispbreads	6.0	0.4
2 tablespoons cream plus water	1.0	0.8
3 sausage patties, 1 ounce each	–	3.0
TOTAL	7.0	4.2

Lunch

	Carbohydrate (*grams*)	Protein (*ounces*)
Mushroom Soup with Parmesan Cheese (page 194)	6.7	1.6
5 ounces sliced turkey breast	–	5.0
Bran-a-Crisp with butter	4.0	1.0
Diet soda	–	–
TOTAL	10.7	7.6

Supper

	Carbohydrate (grams)	Protein (ounces)
Rack of Lamb with Cabernet (page 225)	2.4	6.15
Green Beans with Parmesan (page 243)	10.25	2.3
TOTAL	12.65	8.45

Day Three

Breakfast	Carbohydrate (grams)	Protein (ounces)
Ham and Broccoli Quiche (page 171)	3.1	3.35
1 Bran-a-Crisp with butter	4.0	1.0
TOTAL	7.1	4.35

Lunch

	Carbohydrate (grams)	Protein (ounces)
Clam Chowder (page 195)	5.2	2.15
Pan-fried Salmon (page 232)	–	4.0
2 Bran-a-Crisps	8.0	2.0
TOTAL	13.2	8.15

Supper

	Carbohydrate (grams)	Protein (ounces)
Crab Salad on Belgian Endive (page 186)	10.0	4.0
Roasted Red Pepper Frittata (page 170)	3.84	2.96
TOTAL	13.84	6.96

To nearly any one of these meals you could add as a dessert a ½-cup serving of sugar-free Jell-O brand gelatin (without maltodextrin) or a diet soda popsicle, neither of which would appreciably affect your carbohydrate and protein targets. Again, you're limited only by your imagination, and there are countless different meals you can create that add up to 6 or 12 grams of carbohydrate and the portion of protein you negotiate for yourself.

Remember, however, that the amount of protein for a given meal should be the same from one day to another and likewise, of course, for carbohydrate.

KEEPING A FOOD DIARY

The diary on the following page is an adaptation of a template available in Microsoft Excel. If you're handy with Excel, you can create a daily or weekly plan that automatically adds up the amounts of carbohydrate and protein in the foods you eat at each meal.

You don't need to get that fancy. You can use a piece of paper or just your memory. It's as easy as 6 + 12 + 12. Keeping a record is a good idea, however you do it, because when you find the amount of protein that satisfies you and that also allows you to lose weight if you need to (see next chapter) and to maintain normal blood sugars, you'll want to keep the numbers as steady as possible.

Daily Food Diary

Guidelines
grams carb: bfst-   lun-   din-
ounces pro: bfst-   lun-   din-

Meal	Food Eaten	Carb Grams	Protein Ounces	Comments
Breakfast				
Lunch				
Dinner				
	Total:			

6

Weight Loss — If You're Overweight

Weight loss can significantly reduce your insulin resistance. Obesity, especially visceral obesity (also known as truncal or abdominal obesity), causes insulin resistance and as such can play a major role in the development of both impaired fasting glucose and type 2 diabetes.* Visceral obesity is a type of obesity in which fat is concentrated around the middle of the body, particularly surrounding the intestines (the viscera). A man who is viscerally obese has a waist of greater circumference than his hips. A woman who is viscerally obese will have a waist at least 80 percent as big around as her hips. All obese individuals and especially those with visceral obesity are insulin-resistant. The ones who eventually become diabetic are those

---

*Impaired fasting glucose (or IFG) is treated by most doctors as a sort of "pre-diabetic" condition. They will "watch" it to see if you actually become a diabetic. According to the World Health Organization, IFG is defined as fasting blood sugars over 99 mg/dl. I treat patients with IFG the same way I treat diabetics. For most, it's not a question of if but when they will develop diabetes.

129

who cannot make enough extra insulin to keep their blood sugars normal.

If you have type 2 diabetes and are overweight, it is important that weight loss become a goal of your treatment plan. Weight reduction can slow down the process of beta cell burnout by making your tissues more sensitive to the insulin you still produce, allowing you to require (and therefore to produce or inject) less insulin.

It may even be possible, under certain circumstances, to completely reverse your glucose intolerance. Long before I studied medicine, I had a friend, Howie, who gained about 100 pounds over the course of a few years. He developed type 2 diabetes and had to take a large amount of insulin (100 units daily) to keep it under control. His physician pointed out to him the likely connection between his diabetes and his obesity. To my amazement, during the following year he was able to lose 100 pounds. At the end of the year he had normal glucose tolerance, no need for insulin, and a new wardrobe. This kind of success may only be possible if the diabetes is of short duration — not much damage done — but it is certainly worth keeping in mind. Weight loss can sometimes work miracles.

Before we discuss weight loss, it makes sense to consider obesity, because if you don't understand why and how you are overweight or obese, you will find it somewhat more difficult to reverse the condition.

THE THRIFTY GENOTYPE

When I see a very overweight person, I don't think, "He ought to control his eating." I think, "He has the thrifty genotype."

What is the thrifty genotype?

The hypothesis for the thrifty genotype was first proposed by the anthropologist James V. Neel in 1962 to explain the high incidence of obesity and type 2 diabetes among the Pima Indians of the southwestern United States. Evidence for a genetic determinant of obesity has increased over the years. Photographs of the Pimas from a century ago show a lean, muscular, and wiry people. They did not know what obesity was and in fact had no word for it in their vocabulary.

Their food supply diminished in the early part of the twentieth century, something that had occurred repeatedly throughout their history. Now, however, they weren't faced with famine, because the Bureau of Indian Affairs provided them with flour and corn. An astonishing thing happened. These lean people developed an astronomical incidence of obesity — 100 percent of adult Pima Indians today are grossly obese, with a staggering incidence of diabetes. Fully 65 percent of adults are type 2 diabetics. Over the last several years, even many Pima children have become obese, type 2 diabetic teenagers. A similar scenario is now playing out across the United States in the general population. The pace may be slower, but the result is similar.

What happened to the Pimas? How did such apparently hardy and fit people become so grossly obese? Though their society was at least in part agrarian, they lived in the desert, where drought was frequent and harvests could easily fail. During periods of famine, those of their forebears whose bodies were not thrifty, or capable of storing enough energy to survive without food, died out. Those who survived were those who could survive long periods without food. How did they do it? Although it may be simplifying somewhat, the mechanism essentially works like this: Those who came to crave carbohydrate after having just the slightest bit, and consumed it whenever it was available, even if they weren't hungry, would have made more insulin and thereby stored more fat. Add to this the additional mechanism of the high insulin levels caused by inherited insulin resistance, and serum insulin levels would have become great enough to induce fat storage sufficient to enable them to live through famines. Truly survival of the fittest — provided famines would continue. A British scientist, Andrew Prentice, a professor at the London School of Hygiene and Tropical Medicine, has a theory that Americans in general have a higher incidence of the thrifty genotype. His theory is that people who came to this country through most of its history endured astonishing hardship — a difficult Atlantic crossing that killed off many, then incredible hardship once they were here. Those who survived to have children had to be able to resist that hardship.

A genetic strain of chronically obese mice created in the early 1950s demonstrates quite vividly how valuable thrifty genes can be in famine. When these mice are allowed an unlimited food supply, they balloon, adding as much as half again the body weight of normal mice. Yet deprived of food, these mice can survive 40 days, versus 7–10 days for normal mice.

Recent research on these mice provides some tantalizingly direct evidence of the effect a thrifty genotype can have upon physiology. In normal mice, a hormone called leptin is produced in the fat cells (also a hormone human fat cells produce, with apparently similar effect). The hormone tends to inhibit overeating, speed metabolism, and act as a modulator of body fat. A genetic "flaw" causes the obese mice to make a less effective form of leptin. In recent experiments, when injected with the real thing they almost instantly slimmed down. Not only did they eat less but they lost as much as 40 percent of their body weight, their metabolism sped up, and they became much more active. Many were diabetic, but their loss of weight (and the change in the ratio of fat to lean body mass) reversed or even "cured" their diabetes. Normal mice injected with leptin also ate less, became more active, and lost weight, though not nearly as much. Research on humans has not advanced sufficiently to provide conclusive evidence that the mechanism is the same in obese humans, but researchers believe it is at least equivalent and probably related to more than one gene, and to different gene clusters in different populations.

In a full-blown famine, the Pima Indians' ability to survive long enough to find food is nothing short of a blessing. But when life is almost entirely sedentary and satisfying carbohydrate craving is as simple as nibbling on snack food, what was once an asset becomes a very serious liability. And these people are dedicated snackers. When I visited them and spoke with researchers, I was surprised that they did not keep track of the Pimas' snack food consumption. The response I got was that it was simply impossible because snacking was virtually nonstop. When I saw them off the reservation, they were rarely without a bag of some kind of snack.

Current statistics estimate that slightly more than 60 percent of the overall population of the United States is chronically overweight — and there is even greater reason to be concerned, because the number has been increasing by 1 percent each year since the publication of the USDA's low-fat food pyramid.

The thrifty genotype has its most dramatic appearance in isolated populations like the Pimas, who have recently been exposed to an unlimited food supply after millennia of intermittent famine. The Fiji Islanders, for example, were another lean, wiry people, accustomed to the rigors of paddling out against the Pacific to fish. Their diet, high in protein and low in carbohydrate, suited them perfectly. After the onset of the tourist economy that followed World War II, their diet changed to our high-carbohydrate western diet, and they too began (and continue) to suffer from a high incidence of obesity and type 2 diabetes. The same is true of the Australian Aborigines since the Aboriginal Service began to provide them with grain. Ditto for South African blacks who migrated from the bush into the big cities. Interestingly, a study that paid obese, diabetic South African blacks to go back to the countryside and return to their traditional high-protein, low-carbohydrate diet found that they experienced dramatic weight loss and regression of their diabetes.

It would appear that the mechanism of the thrifty genotype works something like this: Certain areas of the brain associated with satiety — that sensation of being physically and emotionally satisfied by the last meal — may have lower levels of certain brain chemicals known as neurotransmitters. A number of years ago, Drs. Richard and Judith Wurtman at the Massachusetts Institute of Technology (MIT) discovered that the level of the neurotransmitter serotonin is raised in certain parts of the hypothalamus of the animal brain when the animal eats carbohydrate, especially fast-acting concentrated carbohydrate like bread. The next study the Wurtmans performed involved giving students a medication to lower serotonin levels. This resulted in carbohydrate craving.

Serotonin is a neurotransmitter that seems to reduce anxiety as it produces satiety. Other neurotransmitters such as dopamine, norepinephrine, and endorphins can also affect our feelings of satiety and anxiety. There are now more than one hundred known neurotransmitters, and many more of them may affect mood in response to food in ways that are just beginning to be researched and understood.

In people with the thrifty genotype, it may be that deficiencies of these neurotransmitters (or diminished sensitivity to them in the brain) causes both a feeling of hunger and a mild dysphoria — often a sensation of anxiety, the opposite of euphoria. Eating carbohydrates temporarily causes the individual to feel not only less hungry but also more at ease.

COMFORT FOODS AND CARBOHYDRATE ADDICTION

A certain level of this may be true not only of those with the thrifty genotype, but people in general. There's a reason that some foods are referred to as comfort foods. They tend to be high in starch or sugar, and such foods are comforting because they bring about high serum (blood) levels of insulin and high brain levels of an amino acid called L-tryptophan.

Tryptophan is the dietary precursor to the brain chemical serotonin, which is deeply involved in sensations of pleasure and satisfaction. It is the brain chemical affected by the largest number of antidepressants, including Prozac, Zoloft, and Paxil. When insulin levels in the blood are normal, tryptophan has to compete with other amino acids to be admitted into the brain. As such, only small amounts get in. When blood insulin levels are elevated, the competing amino acids get deposited into muscle and other tissues, and tryptophan gets a free ride into the brain. What results is a very power-ful — if short-lived — sensation of bliss, reduced stress, de-creased depression, and diminished anxiety. Comfort food becomes a very easy way to self-medicate, to offset depression or anxiety or stress. When people talk about recreational eat-ing (not in the gourmet sense, but in the quart-of-ice-cream-while-watching-TV sense), they're really talking about giving themselves pleasure by loading the brain with serotonin.

A frequent television sitcom scenario is the depressed woman who plops down on the couch with a pie or carton of ice cream, a spoon, and the intention of eating the whole thing. She's not really hungry. She's trying to make herself feel better. She's indulging herself, we think, rewarding her-self in a way for enduring one of life's traumas, and we laugh because we understand the feeling. But there is a very real biochemical mechanism at work here. She craves the sugar in the pie or the ice cream not because she's hungry but because she knows, consciously or not, that it really will make her feel better. Contrary to popular belief, the fat in the ice cream or in the crust of the pie doesn't make much of a difference. It's the carbohydrate that will increase the level of serotonin in her brain and make her feel better — if only temporarily. The other effect of the carbohydrate is that it causes her blood sugar to rise and her body to make more insulin; and as she sits on the couch, the ele-vated level of insulin in her bloodstream will take that enor-mous amount of food she's just eaten and help her body pack it away as fat.

When I help patients lose weight, I am usually treating an addiction to the brain chemical surges that result from comfort food. As I've mentioned before in discussing the "phasing" common in many low-carb diets, it's completely counterproductive to help someone through carbohydrate withdrawal in phase one, then hit them again in phase two with the carbohydrate you just helped them get over.

On television the actress may never get fat. But for the real-life woman, high serum insulin levels from eating high-carbohydrate foods will cause her to crave carbohydrate again. If she is a type 1 diabetic making no insulin, she'll have to inject a lot of insulin to get her blood sugar down, with the same effect — more carbohydrate craving and building up of fat reserves. This is the central reason that the Diabetes Diet has no phasing and no treat days.

GETTING IT OFF AND KEEPING IT OFF

There may be many mechanisms by which the thrifty geno-type can cause obesity. The most common overt cause of obesity is overeating carbohydrate, usually over a period of years. If you're overweight, you're probably unhappy with your appearance — unhappy knowing that being over-weight often works against us socially, and unhappy with the dangers that accompany overweight and high blood sugars. Perhaps in the past you've tried to follow a re-stricted diet, without success. Generally, overeating follows two patterns, and frequently they overlap. First is overeat-ing at meals. Second is normal eating at mealtime but with episodic "grazing." Grazing can be anything from nibbling and snacking between meals to eating everything that does not walk away. Many of the people who follow this low-carbohydrate diet find that their carbohydrate craving ceases almost immediately, possibly because of a reduction in serum insulin levels. The addition of strenuous exercise sometimes enhances this effect. Unfortunately, these interventions don't work for everyone.

Reducing Serum Insulin Levels

Another group of type 2 diabetics has a common story: "I was never fat until after my doctor started me on insulin." Usually these people have been following high-carbohydrate diets and so must inject large doses of insulin to effect a modicum of blood sugar control.

Insulin, remember, is the principal fat-building hormone of the body. Although a type 2 diabetic may be resistant to insulin-facilitated glucose transport (the movement of glucose from blood into cells), that resistance doesn't diminish insulin's capacity for fat-building. In other words, insulin can be great at making you fat even though it may be, for those with insulin resistance, inefficient at lowering your blood sugar. Since excess insulin causes insulin resistance, the more you take, the more you'll need, and the fatter you'll get.

This is not an argument against the use of insulin; rather it supports the conclusion that high levels of dietary carbohydrate — which, in turn, require large amounts of insulin — usually make blood sugar control (and weight reduction) impossible. I have witnessed, over and over, dramatic weight loss and blood sugar improvement in people who have merely been shown how to reduce their carbohydrate intake and therefore their insulin doses.

Several oral insulin-sensitizing agents, such as metformin, rosiglitazone, and pioglitazone, can also be valuable tools for facilitating weight loss. They work by making the body's tissues more sensitive to the blood sugar–lowering effect of injected or self-made insulin. As it then takes less insulin to accomplish our goal of blood sugar normalization, you'll have less of this fat-building hormone circulating in your body. I have patients using these medications who are not diabetic, and they work in a similar way: the body is more sensitive to insulin, so it needs to produce less, and there is, again, less of it present to build fat. One may also have less of a sense of hunger, and less loss of self-control.

Increasing Muscle Mass

The above suggests what I have been advocating all along — a low-carbohydrate diet. But what do you do if this plus one of the insulin-sensitizing medications does not result in significant weight loss? Another step is muscle-building exercise. The higher your ratio of lean body mass (muscle) to fat, the greater your insulin sensitivity. The better your insulin sensitivity, the less of this major fat-building hormone you have circulating in your bloodstream. Low levels of insulin in your bloodstream mean that more of the food you eat will be metabolized, and that stored fat will "melt away." Chemicals produced during exercise (endorphins) tend to reduce appetite, as do lower serum insulin levels. People who have seen results from exercise tend to invest more effort in looking even better (e.g., by not overeating, and perhaps by exercising more). They know it can be done.

NEGOTIATING YOUR TARGET WEIGHT

Standard formulas and tables are commonly used by nutritionists to determine caloric needs of theoretical individuals — a 120-pound woman who is 5 feet 2 inches tall and exercises moderately needs X number of calories per day. If she's overweight (say 140 pounds), all she has to do is cut her caloric intake so that the number of calories eaten is lower than the number of calories burned. Sounds sensible, like spend less, save more, but it's not. As mentioned previously, if our hypothetical woman cuts her caloric intake too much, she could lose protein (muscle) as well as fat. So she could lose her 20 pounds, but if half of it were muscle, then she'd be worse off than when she started.

Everyone has some level of caloric intake below which they will lose weight. The only way to find out how much food you need in order to maintain, gain, or lose weight is by experiment. Here is an experimental plan you may find useful. This method usually works, and without counting calories.

Begin by setting an initial target weight and a reasonable time frame in which to achieve it. Using standard tables of "ideal body weight" is of little value, simply because they give a very wide target range. This is because some people have more muscle and bone mass for a given height than others. The high end of the ideal weight for a given height on the Metropolitan Life Insurance Company's table is 30 percent greater than the low end for the same height.

Instead, estimate your target weight by looking at your body in the mirror after weighing yourself. (It pays to do this in the presence of your health care provider, because he/she probably has more experience in estimating the weight of your body fat.) If you can grab handfuls of fat at the underside of your upper arms, around your thighs, around your waist, or over your belly, it is pretty clear that your body is set for the next famine.

Your estimate at this point need not be precise, because

as you lose weight your target weight can be reestimated. Say, for example, that you weigh 200 pounds. You and your physician may agree that a reasonable target would be 150 pounds. By the time you reach 160 pounds, however, you may have lost your visible excess fat — so settle for 160 pounds. Alternatively, if you still have fat around your belly when you get down to 150 pounds, it won't hurt to shoot for 145 or 140 as your next target, before making another visual evaluation. Gradually you close in on your eventual target, using smaller and smaller steps.

ESTABLISHING A TIME FRAME

Once your initial target weight has been agreed upon, a time frame for losing the weight should be established. Again, this need not be precise. It's important, however, not to "crash diet." This may cause a yo-yo effect by slowing your metabolism and making it difficult to keep off the lost bulk. I've mentioned it before, but it bears repeating that if you starve yourself, you may lose as much muscle as fat. You will also be more susceptible to going right back to overeating once you've reached your target weight, which may result eventually in your gaining back more fat than you originally lost. This will, of course, increase your insulin resistance and help you get even fatter.

If you look at your diet not just as a short-term means to losing weight (which it will be) but as a long-term means for optimal health, then you'll see that gradual weight loss fits into the Laws of Small Numbers perfectly and makes perfect sense. What you eat when you're losing weight will be essentially what you eat as you're maintaining your weight over the long term. You'll avoid the big inputs (or in this case, big changes) that result in big mistakes.

Thus, I like to have my patients follow a gradual weight-reduction diet that matches as closely as possible what they'll likely eat after the target has been reached.

You'll start the diet, lose weight, and once your weight has leveled off at your target, you'll stay on the same essential regimen you followed while losing weight. "Regimen" is actually an unfortunate word, because it sounds inflexible, but people tend to have the idea that diets are something you do, then stop doing and go back to what you were doing before. This should not be the case. You will get into the habit of eating a certain way, into the habit of eating a certain amount, and over time it will all become second nature.

For this to happen, though, weight loss must be gradual. If your target is to lose 25 pounds or less, I suggest planning on a reduction of 1 pound per week. If you're heavier, you may try for 2 pounds per week. You may find that you lose more than that just by cutting carbohydrate to our guidelines. Don't worry — this has happened to a number of my patients.

Did the paragraph above stop you? You're 25 pounds overweight and if you lose 1 pound per week — Hey! That's six months! And you've probably heard about crash diets on which you can lose that much in one or two or three weeks. You've seen those ads in magazines and newspapers. You're going to a wedding in a couple of months, and no way are you going to fit into that little black dress or that sleek Italian suit. No way do you want to look like a beached whale in the wedding photos. Or bathing suit season's coming up, or your class reunion: 1 pound or even 2 pounds a week is never going to cut it.

If this is the kind of thing you're thinking, then you need to slow down for a moment. Consider first that unless you gained your excess body weight on a crash basis, in preparation for an Oscar-caliber movie role, you're probably like most people and gained your weight the old-fashioned way, slowly — 1 pound here and 2 pounds there. At fifteen or maybe twenty years old, you were perhaps just a little overweight, a little plump — or maybe you were at the absolutely perfect body weight, a svelte, active, fit athlete. But now you're thirty-five or forty. You gained those odd pounds over the years and now it's serious. What do you do?

The best way to lose body fat — and we should really talk about losing fat rather than losing weight — is the same way you gained it: gradually, avoiding the big mistakes.

But what about that reunion or wedding? Maybe all is not lost. The reality is that if you set your target at 1 or 2 pounds a week, it's very likely that you will lose more initially. This has to do with the fundamentals of the truly low carbohydrate diet.

I've seen 350-pound patients whose weight has been trending upward for decades suddenly start to lose more than 5 pounds a week once they follow our low-carb guidelines. Why? Generally these are people who have gained weight because of high intake of fast-acting carbohydrate, which results in chronically high levels of insulin in the bloodstream. They've snacked often, just like the Pima Indians, because they're addicted to carbohydrate and just have to have a little something again and again between meals. They eat just because food is available.

When you get off that kind of food, it's usually not long before you're just not interested. You can walk past the platter of danish or bagels someone has brought into the office. You don't need to keep a drawer full of snacks in your desk at work. You don't snack. You don't overeat at meals. Your meals leave you feeling satisfied, and you're not constantly grazing.

And if you have a rapid goal you want to meet, such as a wedding or a reunion, you can "crash diet" on a truly low carbohydrate diet, although I don't really recommend it. If you understand what you're doing, if you have an idea of the physiology behind why you gained weight and how you can lose it, you can avoid starving yourself and losing lean body mass. In this case, you could considerably trim your protein intake. But keep in mind that a theoretical 150-pound adult needs about 9.5 ounces of protein a day to avoid protein malnutrition.

TRACKING YOUR PROGRESS

So you've negotiated a meal plan with your doctor, following the guidelines laid out in Chapter 5. To offset the low carbohydrate levels in your meals, you are starting out with a protein profile that you think will keep you satisfied. Because weight loss is one of your goals, you have also negotiated a target weight and established a reasonable time frame in which to achieve it. Now it's time to put your plans to the test, to see if they need fine-tuning.

Weigh yourself once weekly before breakfast, and when you do, weigh yourself naked if possible, consistently using the same scale. Pick a convenient day, and weigh yourself on the same day each week at the same time of day. It's counterproductive and not very informative to weigh yourself more often. Small, normal variations in body weight occur from day to day and can be frustrating if you misinterpret them. Generally speaking, most people won't lose or gain a pound of body fat in a day. Continue on your low-carbohydrate diet, with enough protein foods to keep you comfortable.

Weigh yourself after one week, and if you've lost the pound (or whatever your weekly goal is), don't change anything. If you haven't lost the pound, reduce the protein at breakfast, lunch, or dinner by one-third. You can pick which meal to cut. For example, if you've been eating 6 ounces of fish or meat at dinner every day, cut it to 4 ounces. Check your weight one week later. If you have lost a pound, don't change anything. If you haven't, cut the protein at another meal by one-third. If you haven't lost the pound in the subsequent week, cut the protein by one-third in the one remaining meal. Keep doing this, week by week, until you are losing at the target rate. Never add back any protein that you have cut out, even if you subsequently lose 2 or 3 pounds in a week.

If you've managed to lose at least 1 pound weekly for many weeks but then your weight levels off and you want to lose more, you might talk to your physician about special insulin resistance–lowering medications. If it levels off and you've hit your target weight — and a visual inspection confirms you're where you want to be — then you've got your lifetime diet.

If you still need to lose weight, you can just start cutting protein again. Continue this until you reach your initial target or until your visual evaluation of excess body fat tells you that further weight loss isn't necessary. As mentioned above, the average nonpregnant, sedentary adult with an ideal body weight of 150 pounds requires about 9.5 ounces of high-quality protein food (i.e., 57 grams of pure protein) daily to prevent protein malnutrition. It is therefore unwise to cut your protein intake much below this level (adjusted for your own ideal body weight). If you exercise strenuously and regularly, you may need much more protein than this. Once you've reached your target weight, do not add back any food. If your weight falls below your final target, add back some protein.

FINAL NOTES

If You Have Diabetes

While you're losing weight, keep checking blood sugars at least 4 times daily, at least 2 days a week. If they consistently drop below your target value for even a few days, advise your physician immediately. It will probably be necessary to reduce the doses of any blood sugar–lowering medications you may be taking. *Keeping track of your blood sugar levels as you eat less and lose weight is essential for the prevention of excessively low blood sugars.*

The Potential for Blood Clots During Weight Loss

During weight loss, many people unknowingly experience increased clumping of the small particles in the blood (platelets) that form clots. This can increase the risk of heart attack or stroke. Your physician may therefore want you to take an 80 mg chewable aspirin once daily to reduce this tendency. The aspirin should be chewed midway through a meal to reduce the possibility of irritation to the stomach or intestines.

Alternatively, you can use vitamin E in the form of gamma tocopherol or mixed tocopherols. The dosing would

146

be 400 mg 1–3 times daily depending upon your size. It need not be taken during meals like aspirin, as it won't irritate your gastrointestinal tract.

Elevated Triglycerides During Weight Loss

When you're losing weight, fat is "mobilized" for oxidation — i.e., to be burned — and it will appear in the bloodstream as triglycerides. If you see elevated serum triglyceride levels as you're losing weight, it's not something to worry about. Your triglyceride levels will drop as soon as weight loss levels off.

Supplemental Calcium May Help

There is recent evidence that calcium supplements (1,000–3,000 mg daily) may facilitate weight loss by inhibiting the accompanying slowdown in metabolism that may occur when you lose weight. I recommend calcium supplements that also contain vitamin D, magnesium, and manganese. This supplement has also been used to successfully treat the dysphoric mood and carbohydrate craving in women who suffer from premenstrual syndrome.

PART TWO

Low-Carbohydrate Recipes

7

112 Recipes for Low-Carb Meals

The recipes that follow are wonderful examples of how you can eat well with no fast-acting and very little total carbohydrate. While developing a meal plan is a science, it is also an art. The science offers you the metabolic and nutritional underpinnings of what should and should not be in your meal plan. The art portion is the negotiation that has to take place between you and your physician, and between your nutritional needs and your lifestyle, especially your tastes and the time you have to spend in cooking. You can do well with these recipes, but you can also do well by adjusting these recipes to your own tastes. The recipes were developed by Marcia Miele, the mother of a type 1 diabetic, as noted before. Marcia comes from a cooking family. She is an award-winning chef with a fine figure who owns and runs, with her sister Gloria and mother, Daisy, the Peter Herdic House, an elegant gourmet restaurant in a beautiful restored Victorian mansion, situated on Williamsport, Pennsylvania's historic Millionaire's Row. When it comes to food, she knows her stuff. You'll find the low-carb recipes here invitingly delicious and inventive. Her son is fortunate — we should all be so lucky as to have some-one around the house who can whip up dazzling feasts that happen to be good for you.

USING THE RECIPES

All the recipes are, in one sense, a guide to how you can in-corporate foods you may not have considered eating into your diet, and how you can use low-carbohydrate foods and protein to arrive at tasty alternatives to foods from the high-carbohydrate world. (The Parmesan-Crusted Lamb Chops and Parmesan-Crusted Zucchini, for instance, will satisfy your desire for fried food without slapping you with a lot of unwanted carbohydrate.)

You can use the recipes exactly as written and trust that they will play a significant role in assisting you with blood sugar normalization, or you can play with them and cus-tomize them, to suit your own tastes and dietary guidelines. It is best, however, unless you are a seasoned cook yourself, to try the recipes first as they are written and then adjust them to taste. Changes in herbs and spices are generally not likely to alter blood sugars significantly. Including *slightly* more or less protein is fine — this should be part of your negotiation with yourself — but if you're diabetic and tak-ing blood sugar–lowering medication, you will need to ac-count for it. You also need to be consistent from day to day and meal to meal (if you eat 5 ounces of protein for break-fast, then you should eat 5 ounces for breakfast every day).

In general, however, you should follow carbohydrate and protein content guidelines and check your blood sugar to make sure that it remains stable. If a recipe calls for less carbohydrate than required by your meal plan, add some vegetables, salad, bran crackers, or other acceptable food, to the meal to make up the difference.

If you flipped straight to these recipes without learning how a meal plan works, take a look at "Creating Your Own Meal Plans" (page 118) to get a good idea of what makes up a Diabetes Diet meal. Also look closely at "No-No's in a Nutshell," on pages 58–61. It's likely that any vegetable not listed there is suitably low in fast-acting carbohydrate. Remember that ⅔ cup of cooked low-carbohydrate vegetable (or ¼ cup mashed) is *approximately* equivalent in blood sugar effect to 6 grams carbohydrate, as is 1 cup of mixed salad.

NOTES ON THE RECIPES

CHO and PRO

Throughout these recipes the abbreviation CHO is used for carbohydrate (CHO stands for carbon, hydrogen, and oxygen, the elements that make up carbohydrates) and PRO for protein. Each recipe shows the number of servings provided and the approximate grams of carbohydrate and ounces of protein in each serving. (If you are adapting these recipes or creating your own and consulting food value books, remember our rule of thumb, that to convert *grams* of protein to *ounces* of a protein food, you divide by 6.)

Substitutions

Each of these recipes is part of a great meal. You can feel free as you go to substitute one food for another (if you like, say, cheddar cheese better than mozzarella, or olives better than bell peppers). Just remember to adjust the carbohydrate and protein content of the counts in the meal if necessary. You can use the food guide books on page 52, or you can use the USDA's handy calculator if you have a personal digital assistant or a Windows computer (download at www.nal. usda.gov/fnic/foodcomp/srch/search.htm). Don't forget to read the nutrition labels on the packaged foods you buy; see "Nutrition Facts 101," page 95, to brush up on how to read and interpret them.

No Reduced-Fat Products
The recipes use only full-fat ingredients, especially dairy products. Whole-milk versions of yogurt, ricotta cheese, sour cream, and so on are lower in carbohydrate than skim-milk, low-fat, or no-fat versions. Compare the nutrition facts labels at the grocery store and you will see that the differences can be dramatic. This applies to mayonnaise used in the recipes as well.

Measurements
All of the measurements in the recipes are standard American weights and measures. In addition, all oven temperatures are in degrees Fahrenheit.

Chef's Tip
You will note that many of these recipes call for the zest of citrus fruits and grated Parmesan cheese. Some of the best tools you can find for making zest are the Microplane brand of graters. Unlike conventional graters, which use a rasplike

burr, the Microplane series uses a grid of sharp planing teeth. In addition to being excellent for zesting, they also give you very fluffy (and fast) grated cheese.

Da Vinci Syrups

The recipes also use Da Vinci brand sugar-free syrups quite liberally. Da Vinci syrups can be purchased at some health food stores, online at www.davincigourmet.com, or by phone at 800-640-6779.

Using Sugar-Free Sweeteners in Recipes

As you know, the paper packets containing granulated, so-called sugar-free sweeteners usually contain about 96 percent glucose or another sugar, making them inappropriate for diabetics. You can prepare your own granulated sweetener for use in recipes by crushing or grinding aspartame or saccharin *tablets* (not packets) in one of the following ways:

- in a mortar and pestle
- between two spoons
- in a pepper mill
- in a small electric coffee grinder

You can also dissolve the crushed tablets in a small amount of hot water (unless the recipe calls for powdered sweetener).

Aspartame (but not saccharin or cyclamate) will lose its taste if added to food before cooking, so it must be used only after cooking. You may prefer to use stevia, since it is sold as powder or liquid and is not degraded by heat.

Nonsugar sweeteners are not as predictable as sugar and vary considerably from product to product, so it is important to read the package information to verify their sweetening power. When using such sweeteners, sweeten, mix, and sample until you feel you have the flavor you desire. Use only white stevia powder, not green or brown.

Breakfast Dishes

SALMON AND SPINACH OMELET

1 serving   *Per serving: 4.5 gm CHO, 3.8 oz PRO*

	CHO (gm)	PRO (gm)
2 Tbsp butter or olive oil	—	—
1 tsp chopped shallot	0.3	0.1
½ cup chopped fresh spinach	2.0	1.0
1½ oz salmon, fresh or smoked	—	9.0
Salt and black pepper to taste	—	—
2 eggs	1.2	12.0
2 Tbsp sour cream	1.0	0.8
1 tsp chopped chives	—	—

Melt 1 tablespoon butter or olive oil in small skillet. Sauté shallots briefly. Add spinach and salmon. Sauté until spinach is wilted and salmon is cooked. Season with salt and pepper. Remove from heat.

Break eggs into a bowl. Whisk with about 1 teaspoon water. Season eggs with salt and pepper. Melt remaining butter or olive oil in larger, nonstick skillet. Pour eggs into skillet. Turn heat to medium low and cook without stirring. When eggs start to bubble up, place spinach and salmon on one half of omelet. Add sour cream and chives. When most of the liquid egg has set, fold other half of omelet over filling and serve.

SHRIMP AND SOUR CREAM OMELET

1 serving   *Per serving: 4 gm* CHO, *4 oz* PRO

	CHO (gm)	PRO (gm)
5 medium shrimp (41–50 per pound), peeled and deveined	0.5	10.8
2 Tbsp butter	—	—
1 tsp finely chopped shallot	0.3	0.1
2 Tbsp sour cream	1.0	0.8
1 Tbsp scallion, sliced or chopped	0.5	0.12
1 tsp fresh dill	—	—
1 tsp grated lemon zest	0.2	—
¼ tsp paprika	0.3	0.1
Dash of cayenne pepper	—	—
Salt and black pepper to taste	—	—
2 eggs	1.2	12.0
1 Tbsp olive oil	—	—

To make filling, cut shrimp into large pieces. Melt 1 tablespoon butter in small skillet. Add shrimp and shallot. Sauté until shrimp is done, about 5 minutes. Turn off heat. Add next 6 ingredients (sour cream through cayenne) and stir to blend. Taste. Season with salt and pepper.

Break 2 eggs into a bowl. Whisk with 1 teaspoon water and salt and pepper to taste. Melt remaining butter with the oil in nonstick skillet. Add egg mixture, turn heat to low, and cook without stirring. When eggs begin to bubble up, put filling on one half. When most of the liquid egg has set, fold other half of omelet over filling and serve.

WESTERN OMELET

1 serving   *Per serving: 3.9 gm* CHO, *3.06 oz* PRO

	CHO (gm)	PRO (gm)
2 tsp butter	—	—
2 tsp olive oil	—	—
1 tsp chopped shallot	0.3	0.1
¼ green or red bell pepper, chopped	1.9	0.25
½ oz baked ham, chipped or chopped finely	—	3.0
1 tsp parsley	—	—
Black pepper to taste	—	—
2 eggs	1.2	12.0
Salt and black pepper to taste	—	—
½ oz cheddar cheese, grated (about 2 Tbsp)	0.5	3.0

In small skillet, melt 1 teaspoon butter and 1 teaspoon oil. Sauté shallots and peppers until they are soft. Add ham and parsley. Sauté briefly to warm ham. Season with pepper. Remove from heat.

In larger nonstick skillet, melt remaining 1 teaspoon butter and 1 teaspoon oil over low heat. Break eggs into a bowl. Whisk eggs with 1 teaspoon water and salt and pepper. Pour mixture into skillet. Keep heat low. Cook eggs without stirring until they begin to bubble up, 4–5 minutes. Place ham mixture and grated cheese on one half of omelet. When most of the liquid egg has set, fold other half over filling to close omelet. Cook briefly to melt cheese. Serve.

POACHED EGGS WITH ARTICHOKE BOTTOMS AND HOLLANDAISE

4 servings	*Per serving: 6.3 gm* CHO, *2.35 oz* PRO
2 servings	*Per serving: 12.6 gm* CHO, *4.7 gm* PRO

	CHO (gm)	PRO (gm)
1 Tbsp olive oil	—	—
4 oz Canadian bacon, in 4 slices	—	24.0
4 artichoke bottoms	18.0	6.0
Handful of baby spinach leaves, about		
1 cup	4.0	2.0
Salt and black pepper to taste	—	—
½ cup Hollandaise Sauce (page 250)	0.8	0.6
4 eggs	2.4	24.0
1 tsp vinegar	—	—

Heat olive oil in skillet. Sauté Canadian bacon, browning on both sides. Remove from pan and keep warm. Add artichoke bottoms to pan and sauté, stirring artichokes to absorb meat flavor. Add spinach leaves and stir until wilted. Season with salt and pepper. Remove from pan and keep warm with Canadian bacon.

Make Hollandaise Sauce according to recipe on page 250. Keep warm over water bath.

Poach eggs: Put 2 inches of water into a skillet. Add 1 teaspoon vinegar. Bring to a rolling boil. Turn down heat slightly to a lively simmer. Crack 1 egg into a bowl. Holding bowl as close to water level as possible, slide egg into water. Repeat with other eggs. Cook about 3 minutes, or until pink on top. Remove with slotted spoon and season with salt and pepper.

To serve, divide spinach and artichoke bottoms be-
tween two plates. Top each artichoke bottom with a slice of
Canadian bacon and a poached egg. Spoon 2 tablespoons
Hollandaise Sauce over each egg.

RICOTTA PIE

This recipe is a variation of the Italian Easter Pie that my aunt used to make. We eat it for breakfast, or for lunch with a salad. If serving for lunch, you could add 1 ounce each of ham and pepperoni to the pie or add protein to the salad.

6 servings   *Per serving: 3 gm* CHO, *3.8 oz* PRO

	CHO (gm)	PRO (gm)
3 eggs	1.8	18.0
½ cup grated Parmesan cheese	2.0	21.8
15 oz whole-milk ricotta cheese	14.0	49.0
¼ lb diced ham	—	24.0
¼ lb pepperoni, sliced, with casing removed	—	24.0
Butter to grease pan	—	—

Preheat oven to 350°F.

Break eggs into a bowl and beat. Add cheeses, ham, and pepperoni. Mix well. Pour into a 9-inch buttered pie pan. Bake for about 55 minutes.

BROCCOLI-CHEDDAR BRUNCH

4 servings	Per serving: 6.86 gm CHO, 5.23 oz PRO
6 servings	Per serving: 4.58 gm CHO, 3.49 oz PRO

	CHO (gm)	PRO (gm)
4 strips bacon	—	10.0
1 cup broccoli crowns, cut into very small florets	4.0	2.6
¾ lb cheddar cheese, grated (about 3 cups)	12	72
¾ cup heavy cream	6.0	4.8
2 tsp white Worcestershire sauce	1.4	—
6 eggs, beaten	3.6	36
1 Tbsp chopped basil	0.23	0.13
1 Tbsp chopped parsley	0.24	0.11

Preheat oven to 375°F.

Cook bacon in microwave or on stove until almost crisp. Crumble into pieces. Cook broccoli in microwave about 30 seconds or blanch on stove in a shallow pot of boiling water for 2–3 minutes, or until bright green. Sprinkle cheese in the bottom of an 8-inch baking dish. Spread out broccoli and bacon over cheese. Add half of heavy cream. Stir Worcestershire into eggs. Pour eggs over mixture in baking dish, then pour other half of cream over all. Sprinkle basil and parsley on top. Bake for 30–40 minutes.

QUICK BREAKFAST OMELET

1 serving   *Per serving: 3.2 gm* CHO, *3.33 oz* PRO

	CHO (gm)	PRO (gm)
2 eggs	1.2	12.0
1 oz cream cheese, cut into pieces	1.0	2.0
1 oz cheddar or jalapeño cheese, cut into pieces	1.0	6

Beat eggs and place in a ramekin or small microwave-safe dish. Add cheeses. Microwave 1 minute. Stir to blend egg and cheese. Microwave 1 more minute, or until it puffs up, sort of like a soufflé.

To vary the flavor of this recipe, sprinkle 1–2 tablespoons soy bacon bits into the mix before cooking. (Check label for carbohydrate content.)

BACON AND EGGS

1 serving   *Per serving: 1.2 gm* CHO, *4 oz* PRO

	CHO (gm)	PRO (gm)
4 slices thick-cut bacon	—	12.0
1 Tbsp butter	—	—
2 eggs	1.2	12.0
Salt and black pepper to taste	—	—

Put bacon on paper towel in microwave-safe dish and microwave 3–5 minutes, depending on how crisp you like it. Melt butter in small skillet. Crack eggs into a bowl and mix with fork. Season with salt and pepper. Pour into skillet and cook over medium heat, using spatula to turn eggs as they cook. Serve with bacon.

FIVE-MINUTE OMELET

1 serving   *Per serving: 1.2–3.2 gm* CHO, *2.7–4 oz* PRO

	CHO (gm)	PRO (gm)
1 Tbsp butter	—	—
1 Tbsp olive oil	—	—
2 eggs	1.2	12.0
Salt and black pepper to taste	—	—
2 oz protein (from the list below or another of your choice; figures in list are per ounce)	0–2.0	4.0–12.0

Melt butter and olive oil in a nonstick skillet. Crack eggs into a bowl. Whisk together. Season with salt and pepper. Add 1 teaspoon water. Whisk. Pour eggs into skillet. Turn heat to medium. When eggs start to bubble, put fillings, cut into small pieces, on one half of omelet. When most of the liquid egg is cooked, fold other half of omelet over filling. Herbs, such as 1–2 tsp parsley, basil, or scallions, could be added with filling if desired. The carbohydrate herbs would add would not affect your blood sugar unless you used enormous amounts (½ cup, say)

- Cheddar cheese (1 gm CHO, 6 gm PRO)
- Ham (0 CHO, 6 gm PRO)
- Bacon (0 CHO, 6 gm PRO)
- Cream cheese (1 gm CHO, 2 gm PRO)
- Sausage (0 CHO, 6 gm PRO)
- Blue cheese (0.7 gm CHO, 6 gm PRO)
- American cheese (1 gm CHO, 6 gm PRO)
- Pepperoni (0 CHO, 6 gm PRO)

SCRAMBLED EGGS WITH ZUCCHINI
AND CHEDDAR

1 serving   *Per serving: 6.3 gm* CHO, *3.3 oz* PRO

	CHO (gm)	PRO (gm)
2 Tbsp butter or olive oil	—	—
1 Tbsp chopped shallot	0.8	0.3
¾ cup sliced zucchini	2.8	1.0
Salt and pepper to taste	—	—
2 eggs	1.2	12
1 Tbsp heavy cream	0.5	0.4
¼ cup grated cheddar cheese	1.0	6.0
1 tsp chopped basil leaves or parsley	—	—

Heat 1 tablespoon of the butter or oil in small skillet. Add shallot and zucchini. Sauté until zucchini is nicely browned. Season with salt and pepper. In separate nonstick skillet melt remaining tablespoon butter or oil.

Crack eggs into a bowl. Add cream. Whisk together. Season with salt and pepper. Pour into skillet. Reduce heat to medium low. Allow to cook slightly, then add zucchini. Scrape pan with nonstick spatula to turn eggs and zucchini. When eggs are almost done, add cheese and basil. Turn mixture with spatula to mix and melt cheese. Taste and adjust seasoning.

Lunch Dishes

DEVILED EGGS

12 servings   *Per serving: 1.8 gm CHO, 1.01 oz PRO*

	CHO (gm)	PRO (gm)
12 eggs	7.2	72.0
1 Tbsp Dijon mustard, or to taste	—	—
Mayonnaise to moisten, about ¾ cup	10.8	—
1 stalk celery, minced	1.0	0.5
2 Tbsp chopped shallot	1.6	0.6
Salt and black pepper to taste	—	—
24 small pieces celery leaves, for garnish	—	—
24 green olive slices, for garnish	1.0	—

Place eggs in a nonreactive pan and cover with water. Cover with lid. Bring to a boil. Turn heat down so that eggs are just boiling. Cook for 3 minutes. Remove from heat and hold in covered pan for 15 minutes. Run under cold water to peel. Cut eggs in half lengthwise. Spoon out yolks carefully. Mash yolks with fork or put in food processor. Mix in mustard and mayonnaise. Mix in celery and shallot. Season with salt and pepper. Mixture should be moist and sort of fluffy. Spoon back into egg whites. Garnish with celery leaves and olive slices.

168

SALAMI AND PROVOLONE LAYERED TORTE

4 servings   *Per serving: 5.16 gm* CHO, *4.86 oz* PRO

	CHO (gm)	PRO (gm)
½ lb good provolone cheese, sliced thin	4.8	56.0
½ cup Good Seasons dressing, garlic and herbs, mixed (see Note)	8.0	—
½ lb sopressata or Genoa salami, sliced thin	—	48.0
½ cup Pesto (page 254; or see Note)	7.83	12.73

Put a layer of provolone slices in a pie plate. Brush with dressing. Add a layer of salami, then a thin layer of pesto. Continue layering in this way until you have used up ingredients. Wrap in plastic wrap and refrigerate several hours. Cut into wedges and serve.

Note

You can substitute your favorite Italian dressing for the Good Seasons, and you can use a prepared pesto sauce. Just read the labels and make sure you adjust your carbohydrate and protein counts accordingly.

ROASTED RED PEPPER FRITTATA

4 servings   *Per serving: 3.84 gm* CHO, *2.96 oz* PRO

	CHO (gm)	PRO (gm)
8 eggs	4.8	48.0
½ cup grated Parmesan cheese	2.0	21.8
⅛ tsp salt	—	—
Black pepper to taste	—	—
1 Tbsp chopped parsley	0.24	0.11
1 Tbsp chopped scallions	0.5	0.12
1 Tbsp chopped basil	0.23	0.13
3½ Tbsp olive oil	—	—
1 red bell pepper, roasted (see page 182 for method)	7.6	1.0

Break the eggs into a bowl. Whisk to mix together. Stir in Parmesan, salt and pepper, and herbs. Heat oil in 10-inch nonstick skillet over low heat. Pour in egg mixture. Add roasted pepper strips, distributing evenly. Cook over very low heat until top is set, about 15 minutes. Hold a plate over the skillet and gently invert the frittata onto the plate. Slide the frittata back into the pan, cooked side up, and cook briefly to set the bottom. Slide frittata back onto plate or platter. Cut into four pieces and serve.

HAM AND BROCCOLI QUICHE

6 servings   *Per serving: 3.1 gm* CHO, *3.35 oz* PRO
4 servings   *Per serving: 4.63 gm* CHO, *5 oz* PRO

	CHO (gm)	PRO (gm)
1 cup broccoli crowns, in small florets	4.0	2.6
2 eggs, plus 2 egg yolks	1.8	18.0
1½ cups heavy cream	12.0	9.6
Salt and pepper to taste	—	—
¾ cup grated Gruyère cheese, about 5 oz	0.5	42.25
1 Tbsp chopped basil (optional)	0.23	0.13
8 oz baked ham, in small cubes	—	48.0
2 Tbsp butter, cut into small pieces	—	—

Preheat oven to 375°F.

Precook broccoli in microwave for about 30 seconds. Beat eggs, egg yolks, and cream together. Season with salt and pepper. Stir in grated cheese and optional basil. Place ham and broccoli in a well-buttered 9-inch pie or quiche pan. Pour in egg and cheese mixture. Dot the top with the pieces of butter. Bake for 25 minutes, or until the custard has puffed and browned to your liking. Cool slightly. Run a knife around edge of pie plate before removing pieces.

CHEESE PUFF SANDWICH

1 serving   *Per serving: 5.2 gm* CHO, *3.7 oz* PRO

	CHO (gm)	PRO (gm)
2 slices American cheese, ¾ oz each	1.5	9.0
2 leaves red leaf lettuce	0.5	0.3
1 Tbsp Horseradish Dill Mayonnaise		
(page 263)	0.9	—
¾ oz thinly sliced sopressata	—	4.5
¾ oz thinly sliced baked ham	—	4.5
½ oz sliced provolone	0.3	3.5
2 scallions, sliced up diagonally	2.0	0.5

Place American cheese slices 2 inches apart on freezer paper (parchment paper also works but is more expensive). Cook in microwave for about 50 seconds, until they puff up slightly and are crisp. (Each microwave is different, so watch your cheese puffs the first time you make them to ensure they don't burn.) Place a lettuce leaf and half the Horseradish Dill Mayonnaise on one cheese puff, then layer on the sopressata, ham, and provolone. Add the scallion, the remaining mayonnaise, and the second lettuce leaf. Top with the second cheese puff to make a sandwich.

BUFFALO-STYLE WINGS

4 servings   *Per serving: 0.75 gm* CHO, *3.67 oz* PRO

	CHO (gm)	PRO (gm)
24 split chicken wings, about 14.4 oz	—	86.4
Salt and pepper to taste	—	—
6 Tbsp butter	—	—
6 Tbsp olive oil or other vegetable oil	—	—
2 Tbsp chili powder	3.0	1.8
Tabasco sauce to taste	—	—
Olive oil or vegetable oil to fry, about 1½ quarts	—	—

Wash wings and pat dry. Season with salt and pepper. Melt butter and 6 tablespoons olive oil in saucepan. Add chili powder and Tabasco. Pour over wings. Marinate refrigerated for several hours. Heat 1½ quarts oil in heavy saucepan. When oil is hot, fry wings 4–5 at a time (oil should remain hot). Drain on paper towels and season generously with salt and pepper.

Salads

SHRIMP SALAD

4 servings   *Per serving: 7.8 gm* CHO, *5.33 oz* PRO

	CHO (gm)	PRO (gm)
1 lb shrimp, 41–50 count	4.0	96.0
½ tsp Old Bay seasoning	—	—
1 bay leaf	—	—
1 stalk celery, cut in half (will be discarded after cooking)	—	—
½ tsp kosher salt	—	—
½ tsp whole peppercorns	—	—
2 stalks celery, chopped	2.0	1.0
4 hard-boiled eggs, chopped	2.4	24.0
Mayonnaise to moisten, about ¾ cup	10.8	—
1 tsp Dijon mustard	—	—
1 tsp lemon zest	0.2	—
1 tsp chopped parsley	—	—
1 tsp chopped dill	—	—
Salt and black pepper to taste	—	—
8 leaves red leaf lettuce	2.0	1.0
8 leaves Boston lettuce	2.6	1.6
1 small avocado, sliced	3.5	3.7
½ red bell pepper, sliced into strips	3.8	0.5

Peel and devein shrimp. Combine shrimp with Old Bay, bay leaf, halved celery stalk, kosher salt, and peppercorns and

174

steam 3–5 minutes, or until shrimp are just pink. They should no longer be translucent but will become a little tough if they are overcooked. Remove shrimp from steamer and cool. Chop into large pieces, about ½ inch. Add chopped celery, eggs, mayo, and mustard and mix. Add lemon zest, parsley, and dill and mix again. Season with salt and pepper to taste. Serve on mixed lettuce leaves. Garnish with avocado and pepper slices.

SMOKED SALMON ON CUCUMBERS

4 servings   *Per serving: 4.65 gm* CHO, *3.41* OZ PRO

	CHO (gm)	PRO (gm)
24 cucumber slices, about ¼ inch thick	5.0	1.58
Salt and black pepper to taste	—	—
4 oz cream cheese	4.0	8.0
12 oz smoked salmon or lox, sliced thin	—	72.0
4 Tbsp Horseradish Dill Mayonnaise		
(page 263)	3.6	—
4 Tbsp chopped red onion	2.8	0.4
4 Tbsp capers, drained	3.2	—

Season cucumber slices with salt and pepper. Spread with cream cheese. Divide salmon into 24 pieces to put on top of cucumbers. Garnish each salmon-topped cucumber with ½ teaspoon Horseradish Dill Mayonnaise, red onion, and capers. Add grindings of fresh pepper. Salmon could also be rolled around other ingredients and secured with a toothpick for bite-sized hors d'oeuvres.

ANTIPASTO SALAD

4 servings   *Per serving: 6.15 gm* CHO, *4.1 oz* PRO

	CHO (gm)	PRO (gm)
6 cups mixed lettuces (romaine, Bibb, mesclun)	9.0	3.0
½ red bell pepper, cut into strips	3.8	0.5
2 scallions, sliced	2.0	0.5
4 radishes, sliced	0.6	0.2
½ cup broccoli crowns, cut into small pieces	2.0	1.3
¼ cup Edamame beans, boiled and salted, cooled	4.0	5.0
½ cup Dijon Vinaigrette (page 264)	0.8	—
Salt and black pepper to taste	—	—
4 oz sopresatta, cut into strips	—	24.0
4 oz baked ham, sliced thin, cut into strips	—	24.0
4 oz provolone, cut into strips	2.4	28.0
2 oz pepperoni, sliced or in strips	—	12.0

Toss first 6 ingredients in a large bowl with vinaigrette. Season with salt and pepper. Divide onto 4 plates. Arrange meats and cheese on top of each salad.

LOBSTER SALAD

4 servings   *Per serving: 10.9 gm* CHO, *6.3* OZ PRO

	CHO (gm)	PRO (gm)
16 oz cooked lobster meat, fresh, frozen, or canned	6.0	96.0
4 stalks celery, chopped	4.0	2.0
16 green olives with pimiento, chopped	2.67	—
4 hard-boiled eggs, chopped	2.4	24.0
1 cup mayonnaise, or to moisten	14.4	—
1 tsp Dijon mustard, or to taste	—	—
1 Tbsp lemon zest	0.6	0.1
Salt and black pepper to taste	—	—
1½ Tbsp chopped parsley	0.4	0.2
1 Tbsp chopped basil or dill (optional)	0.23	0.13
16 leaves Bibb lettuce	2.6	1.6
8 Deviled Egg halves (page 168)	6.8	24.24
1 small avocado, sliced	3.5	3.7

Combine lobster, celery, olives, and chopped egg. Add enough mayonnaise for desired consistency. Add mustard. Mix together. Stir in lemon zest. Season with salt and pepper. Stir in parsley and basil or dill. Arrange on 4 plates, lettuce leaves first, then lobster mixture, 2 deviled egg halves, and avocado slices.

AVOCADO, MOZZARELLA, BASIL,
AND YELLOW TOMATO SALAD

4 servings   *Per serving: 4.9 gm* CHO, *3.75 oz* PRO

	CHO (gm)	PRO (gm)
12 oz fresh mozzarella, sliced	12.0	72.0
2 oz prosciutto di Parma, sliced paper thin (optional)	—	12.0
1 small avocado, sliced	3.5	3.7
8 thin slices yellow tomato (optional)	2.48	1.4
8 sprigs basil	1.5	1.0
Olive oil	—	—
Salt and black pepper to taste	—	—

Arrange slices of mozzarella, prosciutto, avocado, and yellow tomato with sprigs of basil on platter. Drizzle generously with good olive oil. Season generously with salt and pepper.

CAESAR SALAD WITH GRUYÈRE CROUTONS

2 servings 　　*Per serving: 5.7 gm* CHO, *2.9 oz* PRO

	CHO (gm)	PRO (gm)
1 anchovy, chopped	—	1.0
1 clove garlic, chopped	0.9	0.2
1 egg	0.6	6.0
Olive oil to thicken, about ½ cup	—	—
1 tsp vinegar	—	—
1 tsp lemon juice	0.4	—
1 Tbsp lemon zest	0.6	0.1
Dash Worcestershire sauce	—	—
3 Tbsp grated Parmesan cheese	0.75	8.2
Salt and black pepper to taste	—	—
2 slices Gruyère, 1 oz each, cut into 1-inch pieces	0.2	17.0
4 cups romaine lettuce, ripped into pieces	8.0	2.0

Make dressing: In wooden bowl, muddle the anchovy and garlic until they form a paste. Break egg into the bowl. Beat egg with wire whisk. When mixture is smooth add olive oil a little at a time, whisking constantly, until the dressing is creamy. Whisk in vinegar, lemon juice, and lemon zest. Add Worcestershire and 2 tablespoons of the Parmesan. Season with salt and pepper.

To make croutons, put Gruyère pieces on freezer paper and cook in microwave for about 30 seconds, or until they are crisp.

Toss romaine with salad dressing. Correct seasoning. Top with remaining Parmesan and Gruyère croutons.

SALAD WITH ARTICHOKES, HEARTS OF PALM, BACON, AND BLUE CHEESE

4 servings   *Per serving: 8.7 gm* CHO, *3.85 oz* PRO

	CHO (gm)	PRO (gm)
8 cups mixed lettuces — romaine, red leaf, Bibb, or mesclun	12.0	4.0
8 artichoke hearts, chopped (come in cans)	8.0	8.0
8 hearts of palm, sliced diagonally into 1-inch pieces	6.4	6.4
2 shallots, chopped	1.6	0.6
½ cup Dijon Vinaigrette (page 264)	0.8	—
8 oz blue cheese, crumbled	5.6	48.0
Salt and black pepper to taste	—	—
8 strips bacon, cooked crisp	—	20.0
2 Tbsp grated Parmesan cheese	0.5	5.4

Combine lettuces, artichokes, hearts of palm, and shallots in a large bowl. Toss with Dijon Vinaigrette. Add blue cheese and toss again gently. Correct seasoning. Divide onto 4 plates. Top with crumbled bacon and Parmesan.

ROASTED RED PEPPER SALAD
WITH GRILLED CHICKEN

4 servings   Per serving: 11.4 gm CHO, *5.9 oz* PRO

	CHO (gm)	PRO (gm)
For the Peppers		
2 red bell peppers, cut into strips	15.2	2.0
6 cloves garlic, peeled	5.4	1.2
2–3 Tbsp olive oil	—	—
Salt and black pepper to taste	—	—
For the Chicken		
4 boned chicken breasts, 5 oz each	—	120.0
Salt and black pepper to taste	—	—
Olive oil for brushing	—	—
For the Salad		
6 cups mixed lettuces	9.0	3.0
½ cup crumbled feta cheese, about 2½ oz	2.5	10.0
¼ cup Kalamata olives	3.0	0.5
¼ cup pine nuts	4.4	4.6
⅙ red onion, sliced thin	3.0	0.7
1 Tbsp balsamic vinegar (see Note)	1.0	—
2–3 Tbsp olive oil	—	—
Salt and black pepper to taste	—	—

Roast Peppers

Preheat oven to 400°F. Toss pepper strips and garlic cloves in enough olive oil to coat, 2–3 tablespoons. Salt and pepper generously. Roast on metal baking sheet for about 45 minutes, or until soft and lightly browned. You will hear them start to sizzle in the oven. Check for doneness to personal taste. (I like them browned.) Remove from oven, cool slightly. Transfer the peppers and garlic cloves, along with their oil, to a container. They can be refrigerated or used at room temperature.

Grill and Cool Chicken

Wash and dry breast pieces. Remove skin if you like. Season with salt and pepper. Brush with olive oil. Broil or grill, turning to brown both sides, 10–20 minutes, or until browned and done as you like. Cool.

Make Salad

Mix together all salad ingredients except vinegar and oil. Add roasted peppers and garlic with their oil. Add balsamic vinegar. Toss together salad. Add enough olive oil to coat ingredients, 2–3 tablespoons. The oil in the peppers adds to the dressing, so don't use too much olive oil. Season with salt and pepper to taste.

To Serve

Divide salad among 4 plates. Cut chicken breasts into strips and arrange on salads.

Note

Although we usually avoid balsamic vinegar because it contains sugar, the small amount of carbohydrate per serving will not significantly affect blood sugar.

MINTED CUCUMBER SALAD

6 servings   *Per serving: 4.6 gm* CHO, *0.32 oz* PRO

	CHO (gm)	PRO (gm)
2 cucumbers, sliced	11.8	4.2
3 Tbsp chopped shallots	2.4	0.9
1 medium scallion, sliced	1.0	0.25
Salt and black pepper to taste	—	—
¾ cup sour cream	7.35	5.48
2 Tbsp minced ginger	2.0	—
1 Tbsp chopped dill	1.5	—
1 Tbsp chopped basil	0.23	0.13
2 Tbsp chopped mint	1.0	0.4
2 Tbsp Da Vinci sugar-free mint syrup, or to taste	—	—
2 Tbsp lemon zest	1.2	0.2
Fresh mint sprigs for garnish	—	—

Combine cucumbers, shallots, and scallions. Season with salt and pepper. Combine next 7 ingredients (sour cream through lemon zest) in a separate bowl and mix thoroughly. Season with salt and pepper. Toss sour cream dressing with cucumber mixture. Taste. Adjust seasoning. Garnish with fresh mint sprigs.

MARINATED CHICKEN SALAD

4 servings   *Per serving: 4.85 gm* CHO, *4.18 oz* PRO

	CHO (gm)	PRO (gm)
2 cups cooked chicken breast, cut into large cubes	—	96.0
1 red bell pepper, cut into ¾-inch cubes	7.6	1.0
½ cup cooked green beans, cut diagonally into pieces	2.9	1.2
¼ cup black olives, cut in half	2.5	0.6
¼ cup stuffed green olives, cut in half	2.0	—
2 scallions, sliced, white and green parts	2.0	0.5
1 clove garlic, minced	0.9	0.2
Olive oil to coat, about ¾ cup	—	—
2 Tbsp red wine vinegar, or to taste	—	—
1 tsp chopped basil	—	—
1 tsp oregano leaves	—	—
1 tsp chopped parsley	—	—
1 tsp capers (optional)	0.2	—
Salt and black pepper to taste	—	—
4 large leaves Boston lettuce	1.3	0.8

Combine all ingredients except salt and pepper and lettuce leaves in a bowl. Toss to mix thoroughly. Season generously with salt and pepper. Marinate refrigerated for several hours. Toss again. Taste and if necessary adjust seasoning. Serve on lettuce leaves.

CRAB SALAD ON BELGIAN ENDIVE

4 servings   *Per serving: 10 gm* CHO, *4 oz* PRO

	CHO (gm)	PRO (gm)
16 oz can jumbo lump crab	8.0	80.0
½ cup chopped scallion, white and green parts	2.4	0.9
½ green bell pepper, chopped	3.8	0.5
½ red bell pepper, chopped	3.8	0.5
1 Tbsp fresh dill, chopped	1.5	—
2 hard-boiled eggs, chopped	1.2	12.0
1 Tbsp chopped parsley	0.24	0.11
Mayonnaise to moisten, about 1 cup	14.4	—
1 tsp lemon zest	0.2	—
Salt and black pepper to taste	—	—
Belgian endive, 2 small heads, leaves separated	3.0	1.0
Additional dill and parsley for garnish	—	—
½ small avocado, sliced	1.8	1.8
Olive oil	—	—

Toss first 7 ingredients together. Add mayonnaise to moisten to desired consistency. Stir in lemon zest. Season with salt and pepper. Arrange on endive leaves. Garnish with dill and parsley and avocado slices drizzled with olive oil and seasoned with salt and pepper.

SALAD NIÇOISE

2 servings	*Per serving: 9.5 gm* CHO, *4.4 oz* PRO	

	CHO (gm)	PRO (gm)
4 cups romaine lettuce, washed, dried, and torn into pieces	8.0	2.0
¼ red bell pepper, cut into slices	1.9	0.25
2 scallions, sliced	2.0	0.5
½ cup green beans or haricots verts, steamed	2.9	1.2
¼ cup zucchini, cubed, steamed (optional)	0.9	0.35
6 Tbsp Dijon Vinaigrette (page 264), or to taste	0.6	—
Salt and black pepper to taste	—	—
6 Kalamata olives	1.5	0.3
2 hard-boiled eggs, cut into quarters	1.2	12.0
6 oz canned tuna in oil	—	36.0

Toss romaine, bell pepper, scallions, green beans, and zucchini with vinaigrette. Season with salt and pepper. On 2 plates arrange romaine, scallions, and zucchini, topping with green beans. Arrange peppers, olives, and egg quarters around sides. Top with tuna. Season with freshly ground pepper.

SALAD WITH SESAME SEEDS
AND CANDIED HAZELNUTS

4 servings   *Per serving: 9.8 gm* CHO, *1 oz* PRO

	CHO (gm)	PRO (gm)
6 cups mixed greens, including mesclun and baby spinach	9.0	3.0
½ red bell pepper, cut into strips, then halved	3.8	0.5
½ cup sliced fennel	1.8	0.55
¼ cup chopped scallions, white and green parts	2.0	0.5
½ cup broccoli crowns, cut into small florets, blanched	2.0	1.3
½ cup Hazelnut Poppy Seed Dressing (page 266)	3.7	2.4
Salt and black pepper to taste	—	—
½ cup candied hazelnuts (see Note)	11.0	10.0
4 Tbsp sesame seeds, toasted	4.0	6.4
4 tsp orange zest	1.75	0.15

Mix together greens, bell pepper, fennel, scallions, and broccoli. Toss with dressing. Season with salt and pepper. Mix in candied hazelnuts. Divide salad among 4 plates. Sprinkle each salad with 1 tablespoon sesame seeds and 1 teaspoon orange zest. Season with freshly ground pepper.

Note

To make candied hazelnuts, use same process as Walnut Sweetmeats (page 275), coating hazelnuts with Da Vinci sugar-free hazelnut syrup before toasting.

TURKEY SALAD

4 servings   *Per serving: 3.9 gm* CHO, *4.57 oz* PRO

	CHO (gm)	PRO (gm)
16 oz cooked turkey, chopped	—	96.0
2 hard-boiled eggs, chopped	1.2	12.0
2 stalks celery, chopped	2.0	1.0
2 Tbsp chopped shallots	1.6	0.6
2 Tbsp chopped scallions, white part	1.0	0.25
Mayonnaise to moisten, about ¾ cup	10.8	—
Salt and pepper to taste	—	—

Mix first 6 ingredients. Season with salt and pepper.

Soups

CHILLED CUCUMBER SOUP

6 servings   *Per serving: 4.3 gm* CHO, *0.5 gm* PRO

	CHO (gm)	PRO (gm)
2 cucumbers, peeled, seeded, and diced	11.8	4.2
2 oz cream cheese	2.0	4.0
2 cups chicken stock, homemade or College Inn	—	2.0
1 cup light cream, or to desired consistency	8.8	6.6
1 Tbsp chopped dill	1.5	—
2 Tbsp chopped mint	1.0	0.4
1 Tbsp chopped basil	0.23	0.13
1 Tbsp lemon zest	0.6	0.1
Salt and black pepper to taste	—	—
1 Tbsp Da Vinci sugar-free mint syrup (optional)	—	—
Fresh mint sprigs for garnish	—	—

Combine cucumbers and cream cheese in food processor. Blend until almost smooth. Add chicken stock. Blend again. Add enough cream to reach desired consistency. Add herbs and lemon zest. Season to taste with salt and pepper. If you like it a little sweet, add syrup. Serve in chilled cups garnished with fresh mint sprigs.

CHESTNUT-SQUASH SOUP

8 servings   *Per serving: 11.7 gm* CHO, *0.3 oz* PRO

	CHO (gm)	PRO (gm)
¾ cup chestnuts in shells, or ½ cup peeled, cooked chestnuts	27.15	1.75
1 small butternut squash, about 2 lb (to yield 3 cups cooked squash)	64.5	5.5
2 Tbsp chopped shallots	1.6	0.6
½ cup (1 stick) butter	—	1.0
6 cups chicken stock, homemade or College Inn	—	6.0
Cinnamon, ginger, nutmeg to taste	—	—
Salt and black pepper to taste	—	—

To roast chestnuts, preheat oven to 400°F. Cut an X through each shell with a knife. Put the chestnuts on a baking sheet and roast in preheated oven for about 20 minutes, or until the shells are curling open at the cuts. Cool slightly. Peel while they are still warm, discarding shells and thin brown skin underneath. Chop coarsely and set aside.

To bake squash, lower oven temperature to 375°F. Cut squash in half lengthwise. Remove seeds and stringy material. Roast, flesh side down, on oiled nonstick baking sheet for about 1 hour, or until skin can be pricked with a fork. Remove from oven and scoop out flesh. Use 3 cups of squash for the soup, reserving any extra for another purpose.

Sauté chestnuts and shallots in butter. Add squash and chicken broth. Puree soup to desired consistency with an immersion blender or food processor. Season with spices, salt, and pepper.

ITALIAN WEDDING SOUP
(ESCAROLE SOUP WITH MEATBALLS)

6 servings   *Per serving: 2.57 gm* CHO, *4.4 oz* PRO

	CHO (gm)	PRO (gm)
For the Meatballs		
1 lb ground beef, veal, pork mixture	—	96.0
1 egg	0.6	6.0
2 Tbsp chopped parsley	0.5	0.2
1 Tbsp finely chopped onion	0.9	0.3
2 cloves garlic, finely chopped	1.8	0.4
¼ cup grated Parmesan cheese	1.0	10.9
Salt and pepper to taste	—	—
For the Soup		
2 stalks celery, chopped	2.0	1.0
1 clove garlic, finely chopped	0.9	0.2
4 Tbsp olive oil	—	—
6 cups chicken stock, homemade		
or College Inn	—	6.0
1 head escarole, chopped	6.0	3.6
½ cup grated Parmesan cheese	2.0	21.8
Salt and black pepper to taste	—	—
To Serve		
¼ cup grated Parmesan cheese	1.0	10.9
2 Tbsp chopped parsley	0.5	0.2

Form Meatballs

Thoroughly combine all the ingredients. Salt and pepper generously. Form into small meatballs, between the size of a nickel and a quarter.

Make Soup

Sauté celery and garlic in olive oil in a large stockpot. Add enough meatballs to just cover bottom of pot (do not crowd). Brown meatballs. Remove from pot and brown remaining meatballs. Return all meatballs to pot. Add chicken stock and escarole. Bring to a simmer and simmer about 15 minutes. Stir in Parmesan. Taste. Season with salt and pepper.

To Serve

Ladle soup into bowls. Top with grated Parmesan and parsley.

MUSHROOM SOUP WITH PARMESAN CHEESE

6 servings   *Per serving: 6.7 gm CHO, 1.6 oz PRO*

	CHO (gm)	PRO (gm)
1 small onion, minced	10.0	2.0
2 cloves garlic, minced	1.8	0.4
2 Tbsp butter	—	—
2 Tbsp olive oil	—	—
1 lb mushrooms, sliced	19.0	14.12
1 Tbsp tomato paste (see Note)	3.0	1.0
4 cups chicken stock, homemade or College Inn	—	4.0
4 oz red wine	2.0	0.24
1 Tbsp Da Vinci sugar-free caramel syrup	—	—
Salt and black pepper to taste	—	—
½ cup freshly grated Parmesan cheese	2.0	21.8
¼ cup chopped parsley	1.0	0.4
4 egg yolks	1.2	12.0

Sauté onion and garlic in butter and olive oil until golden. Stir in mushrooms. Sauté 5 minutes. Add tomato paste. Mix well. Add chicken stock. Stir and add wine and caramel syrup. Add salt and pepper to taste. Simmer 20 minutes.

Reserve 2 tablespoons Parmesan cheese and 1 tablespoon parsley to garnish finished soup. Beat together egg yolks and remaining parsley and Parmesan. Stir egg mixture into soup that is just boiling. Garnish and serve.

Note

We usually avoid tomato paste because of its glucose content, but here it adds only 0.5 gram CHO per serving.

CLAM CHOWDER

6 servings   *Per serving: 5.2 gm* CHO, *2.15* OZ PRO

	CHO (gm)	PRO (gm)
4 strips bacon, chopped	—	10.0
2 stalks celery, chopped	2.0	1.0
¾ cup peeled and cubed zucchini		
(¼-inch cubes)	2.9	1.0
½ cup chopped leeks	6.5	0.4
1 bay leaf	—	—
1 tsp chopped thyme leaves	—	—
16 oz clams, chopped	11.6	58.0
3 cups chicken stock, homemade or		
College Inn	—	3.0
¾ cup heavy cream	6.0	4.8
2 Tbsp chopped parsley	0.48	0.22
2 Tbsp chopped scallions	1.0	0.25
2 drops Tabasco sauce	—	—
1 tsp Worcestershire sauce	1.0	—
Salt and pepper to taste	—	—

Sauté bacon in soup pot until almost crisp. Pour off all but 1 Tbsp drippings. Add celery, zucchini, and leeks to pot and sauté until they begin to soften, about 5 minutes. Add bay leaf and thyme. Sauté briefly. Add clams. Stir to mix. Add stock. Bring to a boil. Reduce heat. Simmer 20 minutes. Stir a little hot soup into cream to warm it, then add warm cream to soup, stirring constantly. Add parsley, scallions, Tabasco, and Worcestershire. Taste. Season with salt and pepper.

CREAM OF ARTICHOKE SOUP
WITH TOASTED WALNUTS

6 servings   *Per serving: 9.6 gm* CHO, *0.9 oz* PRO

	CHO (gm)	PRO (gm)
2 Tbsp olive oil	—	—
2 Tbsp butter	—	—
2 cans artichoke hearts, 14 oz each, drained and chopped	36.0	12.0
4 Tbsp chopped shallots	3.2	1.2
1 clove garlic	0.9	0.2
1 stalk celery, chopped	1.0	0.5
½ cup white wine	1.0	0.12
4 cups chicken stock, homemade or College Inn	—	4.0
1 cup heavy cream	8.0	6.4
Salt and pepper to taste	—	—

Topping

6 Tbsp coarsely chopped, toasted walnuts	7.5	6.7
2 tsp chopped parsley	—	—
2 tsp chopped mint (optional)	—	—
2 tsp chopped celery leaves	—	—

Heat olive oil and butter in medium saucepan. Sauté artichoke hearts, shallots, garlic, and celery until soft, about 20 minutes. Add white wine. Cook a few more minutes. Add chicken stock. Bring to a simmer. Simmer about 15 minutes. Puree soup in food processor. Return soup to saucepan. Add cream. Heat to desired temperature. Season with salt and pepper. Pour into soup bowls and top with walnuts, parsley, mint, and celery leaves.

Crab Meat Variation

6 Servings   *Per serving: 10.3 gm* CHO, *2 oz* PRO

Add 8 ounces jumbo lump crab meat (4 gm CHO, 40 gm PRO to the soup along with the cream.

TURKEY SOUP

6 servings *Per serving: 4.18 gm* CHO, *4.12 oz* PRO

	CHO (gm)	PRO (gm)
1 turkey carcass (about 18 oz of turkey meat)	—	108.0
2 stalks celery, cut into large pieces	2.0	1.0
3 garlic cloves	2.7	0.6
10 sprigs parsley	0.3	0.3
1 bay leaf	—	—
3 qt water	—	—
6 cups chicken stock, homemade or College Inn	—	6.0
1 Tbsp olive oil	—	—
1 Tbsp butter	—	—
2 stalks celery, chopped	2.0	1.0
2 Tbsp chopped shallots	1.6	0.6
2 Tbsp chopped scallions	1.0	0.25
2 cups mushrooms, sliced	4.5	4.4
2 cups spinach, chopped	8.0	4.0
Salt and black pepper to taste	—	—
¼ cup chopped parsley and celery leaves	1.0	0.4
½ cup grated Parmesan cheese	2.0	21.8

Place turkey carcass, large celery pieces, garlic, parsley sprigs, and bay leaf in stockpot with 3 quarts water. Bring to a boil. Simmer uncovered for about an hour, or until reduced by about one-third. Add chicken stock. Simmer for another hour.

In a separate soup pot, heat olive oil and butter. Sauté chopped celery, shallots, and scallions until slightly soft. Add mushrooms and sauté about 10 minutes. Strain stock from stockpot into soup pot, reserving the turkey carcass. Take the meat from the bones and cut it into pieces. Add to soup. Simmer for about 15 minutes. Add spinach and simmer another 5 minutes. Season to taste with salt and pepper. Add parsley and celery leaves. Spoon into large soup bowls and top with grated Parmesan.

Poultry

ROAST CHICKEN WITH HERBS

4 servings   *Per serving: 2.2 gm* CHO, 6 oz PRO

	CHO (gm)	PRO (gm)
3–4 lb chicken (free range if possible), about 24 oz meat	—	144.0
Salt and pepper to taste	—	—
4 cloves garlic, cut in half	3.6	0.8
8 sprigs rosemary	1.6	0.3
8 sprigs thyme	1.6	—
8 basil leaves (optional)	1.0	0.5
Bunch lemon balm	—	—
4 bay leaves	—	—
½ cup dry white wine	1.0	0.12

Wash and dry chicken. Season with salt and pepper. With your finger, make 8 pockets under skin of chicken, 4 on breast and 4 on back. Place ½ clove garlic, 1 sprig rosemary, 1 sprig thyme, and 1 basil leaf in each pocket. Fill cavity of chicken with lemon balm and bay leaves. Cover with plastic wrap and refrigerate for 2–5 hours.

Preheat oven to 450°F. Place chicken breast side up in roasting pan and put in oven. Roast for 30 minutes, then reduce heat to 350°F. Baste with pan drippings every 15–20 minutes. Cook about 20 minutes per pound, until thigh juices run clear, or until thigh registers 175°–185°F on a meat thermometer.

Remove chicken from pan and place on a warm platter. Allow to rest 10 minutes before carving. Place roasting pan with pan juices on burner. Add wine to pan and cook, scraping pan bottom and sides to incorporate pan drippings. If there is very little liquid, add a little water. Simmer for about 5 minutes, or until sauce is slightly reduced and wine does not taste sour. Pour half the sauce over chicken and put the remainder in a small pitcher to serve with the chicken.

FRIED CHICKEN

4 servings   *Per serving: 1.35 gm* CHO, *4.33 oz* PRO

	CHO (gm)	PRO (gm)
8 chicken drumsticks, about 16 oz meat (see Note)	—	96.0
1 egg yolk, beaten	0.3	3.0
3 Tbsp heavy cream	1.5	1.2
2 Tbsp full-fat soy flour	3.6	3.6
½ tsp salt	—	—
2 cups vegetable oil	—	—
Salt and pepper to taste	—	—

Wash chicken. Boil in salted water for 25 minutes. Remove skin. Dry on paper towels. Mix egg, cream, flour, and ½ teaspoon salt together until well blended. Heat oil in saucepan large enough to hold chicken.

Oil should be hot, about 365°F. Dip legs into batter and place in oil (tongs work well for this process). Turn when first side is brown, about 3 minutes. When chicken is browned to your liking, remove from oil and drain on paper towels. You can fry a few pieces at the same time, but the oil needs to remain hot. Season with salt and pepper.

Note

Strips of chicken breast meat or other chicken parts can also be used. Strips of chicken breast (about 1½ inches long) do not need to be precooked.

BARBECUED CHICKEN AND SHRIMP
WITH GRILLED ONION GUACAMOLE

6 servings   *Per serving 4.35 gm* CHO, *4.37 oz* PRO

	CHO (gm)	PRO (gm)
1 stick butter, 4 oz	—	1.0
¾ cup olive oil	—	—
2 cloves garlic, minced	1.8	0.4
3 Tbsp chili powder	4.5	2.7
3 Tbsp fresh lemon juice	3.9	0.3
1 lb large (16–20 count) shrimp, peeled and deveined, tails left on	—	96.0
8 oz chicken breast meat, cut in 1-inch strips	—	48.0
Salt and pepper to taste	—	—
1 recipe Grilled Onion Guacamole (page 260)	15.9	8.86

In a small saucepan, combine butter and olive oil. Heat to melt butter. Add garlic, chili powder, and lemon juice. Wash and dry shrimp and chicken. Season with salt and pepper. Arrange in single layer in two separate glass or ceramic containers, shrimp in one and chicken in the other. Pour butter mixture over shrimp and chicken. Cover with plastic wrap. Refrigerate for 3 hours. Bring to room temperature before grilling. Grill over medium heat, turning when brown on one side. Grilling takes 15–20 minutes for chicken, less for shrimp. Serve with Grilled Onion Guacamole.

PEANUT CHICKEN STIR-FRY

2 servings   Per serving: 13 gm CHO, *5.6 gm* PRO

	CHO (gm)	PRO (gm)
8 oz chicken breast meat	—	48.0
Salt and black pepper to taste	—	—
2 Tbsp soy sauce	—	4.0
2 Tbsp peanut butter	6.0	8.0
Dash crushed dried red pepper	0.3	—
1 Tbsp minced ginger	1.0	—
1 tsp Da Vinci sugar-free hazelnut syrup	—	—
2 Tbsp olive or peanut oil	—	—
1 clove garlic, minced	0.9	0.2
⅙ red onion, thinly sliced	3.0	0.7
1 red bell pepper, cut into strips	7.6	1.0
1 cup quartered mushrooms	2.3	2.2
1 cup broccoli crowns, cut into small florets	4.0	2.6
Black pepper to taste	—	—
1 Tbsp chopped parsley	0.24	0.11
1 Tbsp chopped scallions	0.5	0.1
1 tsp lemon zest	0.2	—

Wash and dry chicken. Season with salt and pepper. Cut into chunks for stir-frying. Set aside. In a bowl, blend soy sauce, peanut butter, red pepper flakes, ginger, and syrup, adding a tablespoon or so of hot water if necessary so sauce is smooth. Set aside.

Heat oil in large skillet. Add garlic and chicken. Sauté over medium heat, turning and stirring frequently, until chicken begins to brown. Add red onion, bell pepper, and mushrooms. Sauté until vegetables begin to get soft, 6–10 minutes. Add broccoli. Sauté until vegetables are desired doneness. Add reserved soy sauce mixture, stirring to blend ingredients. Season with black pepper and add parsley, scallions, and lemon zest. If sauce appears too thick, stir in a little water.

Tofu Variation

2 servings   *Per serving: 13 gm* CHO, *2.9 oz* PRO

In place of chicken use 6 ounces extra firm tofu (2 gm CHO, 16 gm PRO), drained and cut into cubes. Omit ¼ red bell pepper. Sauté tofu. Remove from pan. Sauté vegetables, add sauce, then add cooked tofu.

CHICKEN WITH MUSHROOMS
IN A CHAMPAGNE CREAM SAUCE

2 servings   *Per serving: 2.78 gm* CHO, *4.43 oz* PRO

	CHO (gm)	PRO (gm)
2 boneless, skinless chicken breasts, 4 oz each	—	48.0
Salt and black pepper to taste	—	—
2 Tbsp clarified butter (see Note)	—	—
1 tsp minced shallot	0.3	0.1
½ cup sliced mushrooms	1.6	1.1
¼ cup champagne or dry sparkling wine	1.0	0.12
¼ cup chicken stock, homemade or College Inn	—	0.25
2 oz heavy cream	2.0	1.6
1 Tbsp sliced and blanched almonds, toasted	0.66	2.0

Wash and dry chicken breasts. Pound briefly with a meat mallet to tenderize. Season with salt and pepper. Heat butter in skillet large enough to hold both breasts. Add chicken. Brown on one side, then turn over and brown the other side. Remove from pan and keep warm. Add shallots and mushrooms to skillet and sauté until slightly browned. Deglaze pan with champagne, stirring to loosen pan drippings. Bring to a simmer, reduce slightly, then add chicken stock. Again bring to a simmer, and reduce by half. Add heavy cream, stirring. Return to a simmer, reduce slightly to thicken. Season with salt and pepper. Pour sauce over chicken, top with toasted almonds, and serve.

Note

Clarify butter by placing it in a warm pan and allowing it to melt. Skim off the butter solids that rise to the top and discard, leaving clarified butter in pan.

CHICKEN AND GARLIC

4 servings   *Per serving: 4.8 gm* CHO, *4.43 oz* PRO

	CHO (gm)	PRO (gm)
4 small chicken breasts, bone in (about 16 oz meat)	—	96.0
Salt and black pepper to taste	—	—
1 Tbsp olive oil	—	—
2 shallots, chopped	1.6	0.6
2 stalks celery, chopped	2.0	1.0
12 mushrooms, quartered (about 3 oz)	2.7	3.0
20 whole garlic cloves (CHO and PRO amounts have been cut in half because most of the garlic is usually not eaten)	9.0	2.0
1 tsp thyme leaves	—	—
1 tsp oregano leaves	—	—
2 bay leaves	—	—
1½ cups dry white wine	3.0	0.36
3 cups chicken stock, homemade or College Inn	—	3.0
¼ cup chopped parsley	1.0	0.4

Preheat oven to 350°F.

Wash and dry chicken. Season with salt and pepper. Heat oil in roasting pan on top of stove. Brown chicken on all sides. Remove from pan and set aside. Add vegetables and garlic to pan and sauté until garlic is lightly browned. Add thyme, oregano, and bay leaves. Add wine and bring to a simmer. Simmer 5 minutes. Add stock and return chicken to pan. Cover.

Place pan in preheated oven and cook covered for 1

hour. Remove lid. Cook about 20 minutes more, or until sauce is thickened. Remove from oven. Transfer chicken to a platter. Add parsley to sauce. If sauce is desired consistency, taste for seasoning and add salt and pepper to taste. Otherwise, reduce sauce by cooking on stove, then taste and season. Pour sauce over chicken and serve.

CHICKEN WITH FRESH HERBS

6 servings   *Per serving: 1.7 gm* CHO, *5.2 oz* PRO

	CHO (gm)	PRO (gm)
For Chicken		
3 whole chicken breasts with bones and skin on, halved, 5 oz each half	—	180.0
Salt and black pepper to taste	—	—
12 small sprigs oregano	2.0	0.2
12 basil leaves	1.5	0.7
12 sage leaves	1.2	0.6
12 thin slices fresh ginger	1.55	0.2
3 garlic cloves, cut into 4 slices each	2.7	0.6
For Sauce		
1 clove garlic, minced	0.9	0.2
1 tsp minced fresh ginger	0.3	—
2 Tbsp butter	—	—
2 Tbsp olive oil	—	—
1½ tsp Dijon mustard	—	—
1 Tbsp soy sauce (Kikkoman)	—	2.0
2 cups chicken stock, homemade or College Inn	—	2.0
1 tsp chopped oregano	—	—
1 tsp chopped basil	—	—
1 tsp chopped sage	—	—
Salt and black pepper to taste	—	—

Ready Chicken Breasts

Wash and dry chicken breasts. Season with salt and pepper. Lift skin of each breast half along one edge and place 2 each of herbs, ginger, and garlic slices under skin. Cover with plastic wrap and refrigerate several hours. Bring to room temperature before cooking.

Make Sauce

Sauté garlic and ginger in butter and oil briefly, until lightly browned. Add mustard, soy sauce, and chicken stock. Simmer until reduced by half. Add all other ingredients. Taste and season with salt and pepper.

To Finish

Preheat oven to 375°F. Place chicken breasts in a nonstick baking pan and brush with sauce. Bake chicken for about 30 minutes, basting with sauce 2 or 3 times. Transfer breasts to warm platter, bring remaining sauce to a boil, and pour sauce over chicken.

GRILLED CHICKEN WITH PROVENÇAL SPICES

4 servings   *Per serving: 3 gm* CHO, *5.1 oz* PRO

	CHO (gm)	PRO (gm)
2 whole chicken breasts, split, with bone and skin on (20 oz meat)	—	120.0
1 tsp juniper berries	1.0	—
1 whole clove	—	—
1 tsp whole peppercorns	0.9	0.3
¾ tsp kosher salt	—	—
¼ tsp cumin or coriander	—	—
¼ tsp cinnamon	—	—
¼ tsp nutmeg	—	—
2 tsp dried savory	1.5	0.2
1 tsp dried oregano	0.64	0.1
1 Tbsp dried thyme	1.8	0.2
2 cloves garlic	1.8	0.4
2 shallots	1.6	0.6
¼ cup fresh mint leaves	2.0	0.8
¼ cup fresh parsley	1.0	0.4
¼ cup olive oil	—	—

Wash chicken breasts. Pat dry. Grind all dry spices (juniper berries through thyme) in food processor or grinder. Add garlic, shallots, mint, parsley, and oil. Process to a coarse paste. Rub paste on chicken breasts. Cover and refrigerate 3–6 hours.

Bring chicken to room temperature before grilling. Place chicken on hot grill, skin side down. Cook until skin is browned, about 5 minutes. Turn chicken over and cover grill. Cook until meat is completely cooked, about 20 minutes.

ROAST TURKEY

Per 3 oz serving: 0 gm CHO, 3 oz PRO

	CHO (gm)	PRO (gm)
1 whole turkey or turkey breast (as desired)	(See Note)	
Salt and black pepper to taste	—	—
Olive oil to coat bird	—	—
4 oz dry white wine	1.0	0.12

Preheat oven to 375°F.

Wash and dry turkey. Season inside and out with salt and pepper. Rub with olive oil. Place in roasting pan breast side up. Roast at 375° for 15 minutes, then lower heat to 325°. When turkey begins to brown, after about 1 hour, add 2 oz wine to roasting pan. Baste turkey with mix of pan drippings and wine. Roast, basting occasionally, for about 20 minutes per pound, or until internal temperature is 165°F (for white meat) to 175°F (for dark meat). Remove turkey from oven. Baste. Transfer turkey to a heated platter.

Add remaining 2 oz wine to roasting pan. Add ½ cup water. Heat on top of stove, scraping pan to release pan drippings. Reduce mixture until it thickens slightly. Taste. Season if necessary. Baste turkey. Place remaining sauce in pitcher to be served over turkey slices. Chicken stock can be added to pan drippings if you like more sauce.

Serve with stuffing (next recipe) if desired.

Note

Size of bird can vary; turkey meat contains 0 gm CHO and 6 gm PRO per ounce.

STUFFING FOR POULTRY

4 servings   *Per serving: 3.3 gm* CHO, *2.3 oz* PRO

	CHO (gm)	PRO (gm)
1 Tbsp olive oil	—	—
1 Tbsp butter	—	—
4 stalks celery, cut into ½-inch pieces	4.0	2.0
¼ cup chopped shallot	3.2	1.2
¼ cup chopped scallion	2.0	0.5
½ lb loose sausage	—	48.0
1½ cups quartered mushrooms	3.5	3.3
2 Tbsp chopped parsley	0.48	0.22
Salt and freshly ground black pepper to taste	—	—

Heat olive oil and butter in skillet. Add celery, shallots, and scallions. Sauté until celery softens and looks a little clear. Add sausage. Sauté over medium heat, stirring to break up meat, until sausage begins to lose its pink color. Add mushrooms. Continue to sauté until sausage and mushrooms are brown. Stir in parsley. Season with salt and pepper.

Stuffing can be baked inside bird or served hot on the side. If served on the side, spoon a little of the turkey or chicken sauce on stuffing. Makes about 4 cups stuffing.

Beef, Lamb, and Veal

HAMBURGERS (WITH VARIATIONS)

4 servings   *Per serving: 0.4 gm CHO, 4 oz PRO*

	CHO (gm)	PRO (gm)
1 lb ground beef	—	96.0
Salt and black pepper to taste	—	—
1 clove garlic, minced (optional)	0.9	0.2
1 Tbsp chopped parsley (optional)	0.24	0.11
1 Tbsp chopped chives or scallions (optional)	0.5	0.12
1 Tbsp olive oil or butter (if ground beef is very lean)	—	—

If you just want a simple burger, season beef with salt and pepper and form into 4 patties. Add the garlic and/or parsley and chives to the beef mixture if you like an added flavor. Slowly preheat a skillet. Add oil or butter if beef is lean. Sauté patties about 3 minutes per side. Pour pan drippings over burgers.

Wine Sauce for Burgers

4 servings   *Per serving: 0.25 gm CHO, 0 oz PRO*

	CHO (gm)	PRO (gm)
¼ cup beef broth	—	0.1
¼ cup dry red wine	1.0	0.12

When you remove burgers from skillet, deglaze skillet with broth and wine. Mix with pan juices, reduce slightly, and pour over burgers.

Chili Sauce for Burgers

4 servings   *Per serving: 0.87 gm* CHO, *0.12 oz* PRO

	CHO (gm)	PRO (gm)
2 Tbsp Better Than Bouillon chili base	3.0	3.0

Mix chili base with Wine Sauce (above) in skillet until heated through. Pour over burgers.

Cheeseburger

Per ounce of cheese: 1 gm CHO, *1 oz* PRO

	CHO (gm)	PRO (gm)
4 oz cheese — American, cheddar, Gruyère, or blue	4.0	24.0

Place 1 ounce cheese on each burger about 1 minute before burgers are finished cooking. Cover skillet with a lid until cheese is melted.

Herb Butter for Burgers

4 servings   *Per serving: 0.78 gm* CHO, *0 oz* PRO

	CHO (gm)	PRO (gm)
4 Tbsp butter (½ stick)	—	—
1 Tbsp lemon zest	0.6	0.1
1 tsp Worcestershire sauce	1.0	—
2 Tbsp chopped parsley	0.48	0.22
1 Tbsp chopped basil	0.23	0.13

1 Tbsp chopped chives	0.5	0.12
1 Tbsp chopped oregano	0.3	0.1

Beat butter until soft. Add all other ingredients. This can be done in a food processor. Chill slightly, divide into 4 pieces, and place 1 piece on each warm burger.

Mushroom Topping for Burgers

4 servings   *Per serving: 1.63 gm* CHO, *0.2 oz* PRO

	CHO (gm)	PRO (gm)
1 recipe Mushrooms Sautéed with Wine and Garlic (page 245)	6.5	4.72

Serve Mushrooms Sautéed with Wine and Garlic atop or alongside the burgers.

LOW-CARB CHILI

8 servings   *Per serving: 7.15 gm* CHO, *3.24 oz* PRO

	CHO (gm)	PRO (gm)
4 Tbsp olive oil	—	—
2 cloves garlic, finely chopped	1.8	0.4
4 Tbsp chopped shallots	3.2	1.2
4 stalks celery, chopped	4.0	2.0
1 lb ground beef	—	96.0
¼ lb ground pork sausage	—	16.0
2 green bell peppers, coarsely chopped	15.2	2.0
4 Tbsp Better Than Bouillon chili base	6.0	6.0
½ cup red wine	2.0	0.24
½ cup kidney beans	18.0	6.7
2 Tbsp chili powder, or to taste	3.0	1.8
Salt and pepper to taste	—	—
4 oz cheddar cheese, grated (about 1 cup)	4.0	24.0

Heat olive oil in stockpot. Add garlic, shallots, and celery. Sauté briefly. Add ground beef and pork sausage. Cook, stirring to break up lumps, until meat is browned. Add peppers. Continue cooking, stirring frequently, until peppers are soft. Add all other ingredients except cheese. Simmer for 30 minutes, or until desired consistency. Taste and adjust seasoning if necessary. Serve sprinkled with grated cheddar cheese.

POT ROAST OF BEEF

6 servings   *Per serving: 3.3 gm* CHO, *4.27 oz* PRO

	CHO (gm)	PRO (gm)
2 lb chuck roast of beef (yield about 1½ lb)	—	144.0
1 clove garlic	0.9	0.2
2 Tbsp olive oil	—	—
6 shallots, peeled	4.8	1.8
2 stalks celery, cut in ¾-inch pieces	2.0	1.0
½ green bell pepper, cut in 1-inch pieces	3.8	0.5
12 small mushrooms, quartered	3.8	3.7
1 cup beef broth	—	2.0
1 cup dry red wine	4.0	0.48
1 bay leaf	—	—
Salt and pepper to taste	—	—
2 Tbsp chopped parsley	0.48	0.22

Preheat oven to 350°F.

Rub roast with garlic. Heat oil in roasting pan. Brown meat on all sides. When meat is partly browned, add vegetables to pot. When meat is browned, add broth, wine, and bay leaf. Cover and bake in preheated oven about 2 hours, or until meat is very tender. Remove lid for last 20 minutes of cooking process. If pan looks dry, add more beef broth. When meat is tender, transfer to a serving platter. Arrange vegetables around roast. Season with salt and pepper. Season pot liquor. Pour over roast. Sprinkle parsley over all and serve.

TENDERLOIN OF BEEF STUFFED
WITH ROASTED PEPPERS, SPINACH,
AND PINE NUTS

6 servings   *Per serving: 3.7 gm* CHO, 4.42 oz PRO

	CHO (gm)	PRO (gm)
2 Tbsp chopped shallots	1.6	0.6
1 Tbsp butter	—	—
1 cup chopped spinach	4.0	2.0
1 roasted bell pepper, cut into strips	7.8	1.0
2 Tbsp pine nuts, toasted	2.2	2.3
Salt and pepper to taste	—	—
1½ lb piece beef tenderloin	—	144.0
2 Tbsp olive oil	—	—
1 recipe Gorgonzola Sauce (page 251)	6.7	9.3

Preheat oven to 350°F.

Sauté shallots in butter. Add spinach. Sauté until wilted. Add pepper strips and pine nuts. Season with salt and pepper. Butterfly tenderloin, cutting it lengthwise most of the way through so you can open it like a book. Season with salt and pepper. Spread spinach mixture on the inside of the tenderloin. Close tenderloin and tie with kitchen twine. Brown tenderloin in the olive oil on top of stove. Bake at 350°F until internal temperature of beef is at least 130°F, 15–20 minutes. Slice into ½-inch slices and serve with Gorgonzola Sauce.

FILET AU POIVRE

2 servings   *Per serving: 3.6 gm* CHO, *4.32 oz* PRO

	CHO (gm)	PRO (gm)
2 filets mignons of beef, 4 oz each	—	48.0
½ tsp salt	—	—
1½ Tbsp black peppercorns, crushed		
(see Note, next page)	4.0	1.2
2 Tbsp butter	—	—
1½ Tbsp minced shallots	1.2	0.45
2 Tbsp cognac	—	—
2 Tbsp red wine	0.5	0.06
½ cup beef broth	—	1.0
3 Tbsp heavy cream	1.5	1.2

Season filets with salt. Press peppercorns into all sides of meat. Heat butter in skillet. Sauté filets about 4 minutes on each side, until medium rare or to your preference. Transfer to a warm platter and keep warm. Add shallots to the pan and sauté briefly. Add cognac to pan and ignite. (Caution. If you've never done this before, be prepared. The hot pan will vaporize some of the alcohol, and as soon as you put a match to it, you'll get a whoosh of flame. So don't hold your hand over the pan as you're igniting the cognac.) When flame subsides, add wine to deglaze pan. Add beef broth and simmer until reduced slightly. Add cream. Simmer until reduced to desired consistency. Pour sauce over warm filets.

Note

You can crush peppercorns with a pepper grinder on a coarse setting or with a mortar and pestle. If you like a lot of pepper, you can put the pepper on a plate and press the meat into the pepper; if you don't, you can sprinkle on pepper and press it in that way.

PARMESAN-CRUSTED LAMB CHOPS

2 servings   *Per serving: 1.8 gm* CHO, *6.7 oz* PRO

	CHO (gm)	PRO (gm)
8 miniature rib lamb chops, French cut (meat trimmed away from end of bone so that bone is clean), cut singly, about 7 oz meat	—	42.0
Salt and black pepper to taste	—	—
1 egg, slightly beaten	0.6	6.0
¾ cup freshly grated Parmesan cheese	3.0	32.7
Olive oil to fry, about 1 cup	—	—

Season lamb chops with salt and pepper. Dip individually in egg, then parmesan. Fry in oil in skillet. Oil should cover the lamb chops. Oil should be hot, simmering when you insert lamb chops. Fry until crisp, about 5 minutes. Allow them to become golden brown. Drain on paper towels. Season with salt and pepper and serve.

LAMB CHOPS WITH MINT PERSILLADE

4 servings   *Per serving: 1.8 gm* CHO, *4.1 oz* PRO

	CHO (gm)	PRO (gm)
16 baby lamb chops (2 rib racks, cut individually), about 1 lb meat	—	96.0
2 cloves garlic, minced	1.8	0.4
½ cup chopped mint leaves	4.0	1.6
¼ cup chopped parsley	1.0	0.4
2 Tbsp chopped basil	0.46	0.26
1 Tbsp kosher salt	—	—
Black pepper to taste	—	—

Separate lamb chops. Mix garlic and herbs and chop to-gether briefly. Mix in salt and pepper. Rub mixture all over chops. Grill over medium-high heat until outside is crisp, 5–10 minutes on each side.

Note
Persil is French for parsley, and persillade indicates a unique mix of parsley and garlic or shallots.

RACK OF LAMB WITH CABERNET

1 serving	*Per serving: 2.4 gm* CHO, *6.15 oz* PRO

	CHO (gm)	PRO (gm)
6 miniature rib lamb chops, French cut (meat trimmed away from end of bone so that bone is clean), cut into 2-rib sections, about 6 oz meat	—	36.0
Salt and black pepper to taste	—	—
1 clove garlic, split (optional, to rub lamb)	—	—
½ Tbsp shallots	0.4	0.15
½ cup cabernet or other dry red wine	2.0	0.24
¼ cup beef stock	—	0.5
2 Tbsp cold butter, cut into pieces	—	—

Wash and dry lamb chops, season with salt and pepper, and rub with garlic clove if you like. Set aside while you make the sauce.

Put shallots, cabernet, and beef stock in a small saucepan. Bring to a boil, turn heat down, and simmer until sauce is reduced by half. Turn heat off and stir in cold butter pieces to thicken. Keep warm. Broil or grill lamb chops, turning to brown all sides, to desired doneness, 5–10 minutes. Serve with sauce.

VEAL WITH FENNEL AND WILD MUSHROOMS
IN MUSTARD CREAM

4 servings *Per serving: 5 gm* CHO, *4.5 oz* PRO

	CHO (gm)	PRO (gm)
16 oz veal scallops	—	96.0
Salt and black pepper to taste	—	—
1 Tbsp olive oil	—	—
1 Tbsp butter	—	—
1 clove garlic, minced	0.9	0.2
1 Tbsp minced shallots	0.8	0.3
8 oz mixed mushrooms — enoki, oyster, button, or other — sliced	9.5	7.0
½ cup thinly sliced fennel	1.8	0.55
½ cup chardonnay	1.0	0.12
¾ cup heavy cream	6.0	4.8
½ tsp Dijon mustard	—	—

Pound veal scallops lightly with meat mallet. Season with salt and pepper. Sauté veal in skillet in oil and butter in single layer. As scallops brown, remove them from pan and place on a warm platter. Keep warm while you make the sauce.

Add garlic, shallots, mushrooms, and fennel to pan. Sauté until vegetables begin to brown. Add chardonnay and simmer until wine is reduced by a third. Add cream and mustard and simmer until sauce reduces slightly and thickens. Taste and adjust seasoning if necessary. Spoon sauce over veal scallops.

Pork

BAKED PORK CHOPS

4 servings   *Per serving: 1.3 gm CHO, 4 oz PRO*

	CHO (gm)	PRO (gm)
4 center-cut pork chops, with bone, 4 oz of meat each	—	96.0
2 cloves garlic	1.8	0.4
4 large sprigs rosemary	0.8	—
Salt and black pepper to taste	—	—
Olive oil to pan-fry, about ¼ cup	—	—
½ cup chopped basil leaves	1.8	1.0
¼ cup dry red wine	1.0	0.12

Rub pork chops with garlic and rosemary. Season with salt and pepper. Brown chops in oil in a skillet. Chop garlic, rosemary, and basil. When chops are browned on both sides, transfer them to an ovenproof baking dish or pan. Spread chopped herb mixture on the chops. Preheat oven to 350°F.

Deglaze the skillet with wine (water can be used instead). Pour in wine while the pan is still hot and scrape the pan drippings from sides and bottom of pan. Simmer the wine mixture for 5 minutes. Pour over pork chops. Bake chops for about 1 hour.

PORK ROAST WITH ROSEMARY AND SAGE

6 servings   *Per serving: 2 gm* CHO, *5.4 oz* PRO

	CHO (gm)	PRO (gm)
6 cloves garlic	5.4	1.2
¼ cup rosemary leaves	1.4	0.24
6 sage leaves, chopped	0.6	0.3
6 sprigs thyme	1.2	—
¼ cup parsley	1.0	0.4
1 Tbsp coarse salt	—	—
1 Tbsp ground black pepper	2.7	0.9
2 Tbsp olive oil	—	—
1 boneless pork loin roast, about 2 lb (see Note)	—	192.0

Preheat oven to 450°F.

Combine garlic, rosemary, sage, thyme, parsley, salt, and pepper in a food processor. Blend to make a paste. This can also be done with mortar and pestle. Add olive oil. Open the pork roast and spread half of the mixture on the inside of the roast. Roll roast back to its original shape and tie it with butcher's string. Spread remaining herb mixture all over the surface of the roast.

Place roast fat side up in a roasting pan in the preheated oven. Reduce heat to 325°F. Cook about 1 hour, or until the internal temperature of the roast is 170°F. Allow to rest 10 minutes before carving. Can be served hot or at room temperature.

Note

Ask the butcher for a boned and tied roast — but ask him to leave it untied and give you the string. Then tie it yourself once you have spread it with the herb mixture.

PORK CHOPS WITH PEPPERS

This simple recipe is a delicious dinner my mother made when I was growing up, and I make it often now.

4 servings   *Per serving: 5 gm* CHO, *4.1 oz* PRO

	CHO (gm)	PRO (gm)
4 pork chops, 4 oz of meat each	—	96.0
Salt and black pepper to taste	—	—
2 Tbsp olive oil	—	—
4 small green bell peppers, cut into thick strips	20.0	2.4

Preheat oven to 375°F.

Wash and dry pork chops. Season with salt and pepper. Brown pork chops in olive oil in large skillet over medium heat. Add as many peppers as can comfortably fit in the skillet. When pork chops and peppers are nicely browned, transfer them to a roasting pan with a lid. Brown remainder of peppers in the skillet with the meat juices. Transfer these peppers to the roasting pan.

Cover the pan and place in preheated oven. Bake until pork chops and peppers are soft, at least 1 hour. Cooking longer won't hurt. Remove lid for last 20 minutes of cooking if there is more liquid than you like. Taste and adjust seasoning. Serve pork chops topped with peppers and cooking liquid.

MUSHROOMS STUFFED WITH SAUSAGE AND RICOTTA

4 servings   *Per serving: 4.2 gm* CHO, *4.94 oz* PRO

	CHO (gm)	PRO (gm)
24 mushroom caps, medium to large	7.2	8.0
1 lb loose pork sausage	—	96.0
2 Tbsp chopped shallots	1.6	0.6
4 cups spinach leaves, washed, with large stems removed (tear larger leaves into 3–4 pieces)	4.0	2.0
½ cup whole-milk ricotta cheese	4.0	12.0

Preheat oven to 350°F.

Prebake mushrooms on a baking sheet until soft, 15–20 minutes. Pour off liquid. Sauté sausage and shallots in skillet until sausage is cooked. Add spinach and sauté until spinach is wilted. Add ricotta. Stir to mix well. Spoon mixture into mushroom caps. Broil mushrooms briefly to brown, about 5 minutes.

Seafood

PAN-FRIED SALMON

Try serving this salmon with Mustard Sorrel Sauce (page 252) or Aioli (page 253).

4 servings   *Per serving: 0 gm CHO, 4 oz PRO*

	CHO (gm)	PRO (gm)
4 salmon fillets, 4 oz each	—	96.0
Salt and black pepper to taste	—	—
1½ Tbsp butter	—	—
1½ Tbsp olive oil	—	—

Wash and dry salmon. Season with salt and pepper. Heat butter and oil in skillet. Sauté salmon over medium-high heat. Brown one side, then turn over to brown the other side. It takes 6–8 minutes.

SALMON TERIYAKI

6 servings   *Per serving: 0.73 gm* CHO, *4.9 oz* PRO

	CHO (gm)	PRO (gm)
1 cup Kikkoman soy sauce	—	32.0
3 Tbsp Da Vinci sugar-free hazelnut syrup	—	—
½ tsp dry mustard	—	—
2 cloves garlic, minced	1.8	0.4
¼ cup chopped parsley	1.0	0.4
¼ cup dry red wine	1.0	0.12
6 salmon fillets, 4 oz each	—	144.0
4 Tbsp butter (½ stick)	—	—
1 Tbsp lemon zest	0.6	0.1

Combine soy sauce, syrup, mustard, garlic, parsley, and wine. Mix well. Place salmon in a ceramic or glass dish and pour marinade over it. Cover with plastic wrap, refrigerate, and marinate 4 hours.

Remove salmon from refrigerator about 30 minutes before ready to grill. Melt butter in small saucepan. Add lemon zest. Remove salmon from marinade and grill 6–8 minutes, basting with butter sauce.

FLOUNDER WITH SPINACH AND PINE NUTS
IN LEMON THYME BUTTER

1 serving   *Per serving: 6.7 gm* CHO, *4.4 oz* PRO

	CHO (gm)	PRO (gm)
4 oz flounder fillet, bones removed	—	24.0
Salt and black pepper to taste	—	—
1 Tbsp clarified butter (see Note, page 207) or olive oil	—	—
1 Tbsp sun-dried tomato in oil, chopped	3.0	1.0
1 tsp minced shallot	0.8	0.3
2 tsp pine nuts, toasted	0.75	0.76
2 oz dry white wine	0.5	0.06
4 large spinach leaves, washed thoroughly	1.25	0.25
Squeeze of lemon juice	0.4	—
1 tsp fresh lemon thyme	—	—
1 Tbsp soft butter	—	—

Wash and dry flounder fillet. Season with salt and pepper. Heat clarified butter or oil in sauté pan over medium-high heat. Sauté flounder on one side, then turn over to brown the other side. Reduce heat to medium. Add sun-dried tomatoes, shallots, and pine nuts; toss until browned. Transfer flounder from pan to warm plate. Deglaze pan with white wine. Add spinach and cook just until it wilts. Arrange spinach around flounder on plate. Add lemon juice, lemon thyme, and softened butter to pan juices and stir gently. Taste sauce and adjust seasoning. Pour sauce over flounder.

FLOUNDER WITH MERLOT

4 servings   *Per serving: 6.25 gm* CHO, *4.2 oz* PRO

	CHO (gm)	PRO (gm)
¾ cup bell peppers, green or red, cut into julienne strips	6.9	0.9
¾ cup scallions, cut into julienne strips	6.0	1.5
¾ cup celery, cut into julienne strips	1.5	0.75
2 cloves garlic, finely chopped	1.8	0.4
1 tsp chopped ginger	0.3	—
½ cup butter (1 stick)	—	1.0
8 small flounder fillets, about 2 oz each	—	96.0
Salt and black pepper to taste	—	—
½ cup chopped leeks, white part only	6.5	0.4
½ cup dry merlot	2.0	0.24
1 tsp Da Vinci sugar-free caramel syrup	—	—
1 tsp chopped parsley or mint	—	—

Preheat oven to 350°F.

Sauté first 5 ingredients (bell peppers through ginger) in 2 tablespoons of the butter. Season fish with salt and pepper. Arrange 4 fillets on a bed of chopped leeks in a small baking pan. Distribute the sautéed vegetables evenly over the 4 fillets. Cover with remaining flounder fillets. Combine merlot and syrup and add to baking pan. Cover with foil and bake 20 minutes. Transfer fish to warm platter and keep warm. Transfer liquid in pan to small skillet or saucepan. Cook until liquid is reduced slightly. Lower heat and whisk in remaining butter a tablespoon at a time. Season with salt and pepper. Spoon sauce over fish. Garnish with parsley or mint.

GRILLED SWORDFISH WITH ARTICHOKE
AND HEARTS OF PALM SALSA

4 servings *Per serving: 4.2 gm* CHO, *4.3 oz* PRO

	CHO (gm)	PRO (gm)
For the Salsa		
4 stalks hearts of palm, cut diagonally into ½-inch slices	3.2	3.2
4 artichoke hearts, chopped	9.0	3.0
2 Tbsp chopped scallions	1.0	0.25
8 Kalamata olives, chopped	2.0	0.35
¼ cup fennel, cut diagonally in ¼-inch pieces	1.0	0.3
¼ cup Dijon Vinaigrette (page 264)	—	—
Salt and black pepper to taste	—	—
1 Tbsp chopped parsley	0.24	0.11
1 Tbsp chopped basil	0.23	0.13
For the Swordfish		
4 swordfish steaks, 4 oz each	—	96.0
Salt and pepper to taste	—	—
Olive oil to brush fish	—	—

Make Salsa

Combine all ingredients. Set aside for several hours to allow flavors to blend. Salsa does not need to be cooked, but it can be heated in a skillet or microwave if you prefer it warm.

Grill Swordfish

Season swordfish steaks with salt and pepper. Brush with olive oil. Grill or broil to desired doneness, 3–4 minutes on each side. Top with the salsa.

GRILLED SWORDFISH WITH GINGER
ORANGE MARINADE

4 servings   *Per serving: 1.9 gm* CHO, *4.4 oz* PRO

	CHO (gm)	PRO (gm)
2 cloves garlic, finely chopped	1.8	0.4
1 full Tbsp finely chopped ginger	1.0	—
¼ cup sesame oil	—	—
¼ cup Kikkoman soy sauce	—	8.0
¼ cup dry white wine	0.5	0.06
4 small scallions, sliced in rings	2.0	0.5
1 Tbsp Da Vinci sugar-free orange syrup	—	—
Grated zest of one orange	1.5	0.1
Pinch of dried crushed red pepper	0.3	—
¼ jalapeño pepper, minced	0.4	0.1
Black pepper to taste	—	—
4 swordfish steaks, 4 oz each	—	96.0

Mix together all ingredients except black pepper and fish to make marinade. Wash and dry swordfish, place in a ceramic or glass dish, and season with black pepper. Pour marinade over fish and cover with plastic wrap. Marinate for several hours refrigerated or half an hour at room temperature. Turn occasionally to coat fish well.

Remove fish from refrigerator about 30 minutes before ready to grill. Remove fish from marinade and pour marinade into a small saucepan. Grill fish over medium heat to desired doneness, brushing with marinade, 10–15 minutes. Bring remaining marinade to a boil. Pour over swordfish. This marinade also works well with salmon.

SHRIMP WITH MACADAMIA CRUST

4 servings   *Per serving: 5.9 gm CHO, 3.8 oz PRO*

	CHO (gm)	PRO (gm)
20 large shrimp, peeled and deveined, tails left on, 12 oz meat	—	72.0
1 egg, lightly beaten	0.6	6.0
Salt and black pepper to taste	—	—
1¼ cup macadamia nuts, toasted and ground in a food processor	23.13	13.25
Olive oil to make ⅛-inch layer in bottom of skillet, about ¼ cup	—	—

Wash and dry shrimp. Season egg with salt and pepper and put in a shallow bowl for dipping. Season ground macadamia nuts and put on a plate. Heat oil to medium high. Dip shrimp in egg, then coat with macadamia nuts. Fry in hot oil until crisp. Drain on paper towels.

Coconut and Macadamia Crust Variation

4 servings   *Per serving: 5.2 gm CHO, 3.45 oz PRO*

Substitute ½ cup grated unsweetened coconut, toasted (6.2 gm CHO, 2 gm PRO), for ½ cup macadamias. Replace half the olive oil with coconut oil. Proceed as above.

Vegetables

ROASTED VEGETABLES

4 servings   *Per serving: 7.3 gm* CHO, *0.6 oz* PRO

	CHO (gm)	PRO (gm)
1 red bell pepper, cut in strips about 1¼ inches wide	7.6	1.0
1 cup mushrooms, whole or halved if they are big	1.8	2.0
½ bulb fennel, cut in thick triangles	4.9	1.45
20 spears asparagus	8.0	8.0
4 shallots, peeled	3.2	0.9
4 cloves garlic, peeled	3.6	0.8
Olive oil to coat	—	—
Salt and black pepper to taste	—	—

Preheat oven to 450°F.

Toss vegetables with a generous coating of olive oil. Season with salt and pepper. Spread on baking sheet. Roast at 450°F for 15 minutes, then reduce heat to 375°F. Check for desired doneness. Asparagus could be done at this point. I like things browned, so I would cook asparagus about 30 minutes in all and peppers about 1 hour. Check every 15 minutes and remove vegetables that are done to your liking. Rub vegetables in brown pan oil to get flavor. Serve warm or at room temperature, alone or with Aioli (page 253).

240

BROCCOLI WITH GARLIC AND PARMESAN

4 servings   *Per serving: 2.75 gm* CHO, *0.7 oz* PRO

	CHO (gm)	PRO (gm)
2 cups broccoli florets	8.0	5.2
3 Tbsp olive oil	—	—
2 garlic cloves, minced	1.8	0.4
Salt and black pepper to taste	—	—
¼ cup freshly grated Parmesan cheese	1.0	10.9
2 Tbsp chopped basil	0.23	0.13

Cook broccoli in microwave for about 30 seconds, until it is bright green and just a little cooked. Heat olive oil in skillet. Sauté garlic for 2 minutes. Add broccoli. Stir to coat with oil. Sauté 3–5 minutes, until broccoli reaches desired doneness. Season with salt and pepper. Toss with Parmesan and basil.

MASHED CAULIFLOWER

If you love mashed potatoes and can't stand the idea of giving them up, this is a very pleasant surprise.

4 servings   *Per serving: 4.8 gm* CHO, *0.35 oz* PRO

	CHO (gm)	PRO (gm)
½ head cauliflower, tough stem trimmed	15.25	5.7
Salt to taste	—	—
4 oz butter (1 stick)	—	1.0
¼ cup heavy cream	4.0	1.6
Black pepper to taste	—	—

Steam cauliflower until fairly soft, about 15 minutes, adding salt to steamer. Pull florets apart with a fork. Put pieces into a mixing bowl. Add butter and heavy cream. Beat with electric mixer or mash with potato masher. Season generously with salt and pepper. Reheat in microwave if necessary.

Depending on your taste, you can add a small amount of fresh herbs, such as rosemary or chives, to enhance flavor without affecting the carbohydrate portion.

242

GREEN BEANS WITH PARMESAN

4 servings   *Per serving: 10.25 gm CHO, 2.3 oz PRO*

	CHO (gm)	PRO (gm)
4 cups green beans, trimmed	23.2	9.6
½ red onion, thinly sliced	10.0	2.0
½ cup olive oil	—	—
2 Tbsp balsamic vinegar (see Note)	2.0	—
2 cloves garlic, finely chopped	1.8	0.4
1 cup freshly grated Parmesan cheese	4.0	43.6
Salt and black pepper to taste	—	—

Cook beans in steamer until tender, about 15 minutes. Drain. Mix together with onion, oil, vinegar, and garlic. Then add Parmesan, tossing to mix completely. Season with salt and pepper to taste. Can be served warm, cold, or at room temperature.

Note

Although we usually avoid balsamic vinegar because it contains sugar, the small amount of carbohydrate per serving will not significantly affect blood sugar.

MARINATED MUSHROOMS

Other vegetables, such as green beans, zucchini, summer squash, green peppers, and leeks, can also be marinated in this way.

6 servings   *Per serving: 3.9 gm* CHO, *0.5 oz* PRO

	CHO (gm)	PRO (gm)
3 cups chicken stock, homemade or College Inn	—	3.0
1 cup dry white wine	2.0	0.24
1 cup olive oil	—	—
1 small bunch parsley, 10 sprigs	0.6	0.3
2 cloves garlic, pressed	1.9	0.4
1 tsp thyme leaves	—	—
1 bay leaf	—	—
10 peppercorns	—	—
1 tsp salt	—	—
1 lb mushrooms (leave whole if small; otherwise halve or quarter them)	19.0	14.12

Place all ingredients except mushrooms in saucepan. Bring to a boil, reduce heat, and simmer gently for 45 minutes. Strain marinade and return it to saucepan. Bring to a simmer. Add mushrooms and simmer, covered, for about 10 minutes. Transfer mushrooms and marinade to a ceramic or glass dish. Taste marinade and adjust seasoning. Cover dish with plastic wrap and marinate for at least 4 hours. Remove mushrooms with slotted spoon and spoon some marinade over them.

MUSHROOMS SAUTÉED WITH WINE
AND GARLIC

2 servings   *Per serving: 3.25 gm* CHO, *0.4 oz* PRO

	CHO (gm)	PRO (gm)
2 Tbsp olive oil	—	—
1 clove garlic, finely chopped	0.9	0.2
2 cups sliced mushrooms	4.6	4.4
¼ cup dry red wine	1.0	0.12
Salt and black pepper to taste	—	—

Heat olive oil in skillet. Add garlic, sauté briefly, about 1 minute. Add mushrooms. Sauté 1 minute. Add wine. Continue to sauté until all liquid is absorbed, about 10 minutes. Season with salt and pepper.

SAUTÉED SPINACH WITH GARLIC
AND PINE NUTS

4 servings   *Per serving: 4.9 gm* CHO, *0.65 oz* PRO

	CHO (gm)	PRO (gm)
2 Tbsp olive oil	—	—
1 clove garlic, peeled and chopped finely	0.9	0.2
1 lb fresh spinach, washed thoroughly, stems removed if too thick	16.5	13.0
2 Tbsp pine nuts, toasted and salted	2.2	2.3
Salt and black pepper to taste	—	—

Heat olive oil in skillet over medium heat. Sauté garlic until lightly browned, about 2 minutes. Add spinach and sauté until it is all wilted, about 10 minutes. Add pine nuts, stirring to distribute evenly. Season with salt and pepper and serve.

BUTTERNUT SQUASH WITH COGNAC

8 servings   Per serving: 11 gm CHO, *0.2 oz* PRO

	CHO (gm)	PRO (gm)
1 butternut squash, about 2½ lb (to yield 4 cups cooked squash)	86.0	7.3
1½ sticks butter, cut into pieces	—	1.5
2 Tbsp Da Vinci sugar-free caramel syrup	—	—
¼ cup cognac	—	—
1 tsp cinnamon	1.84	0.1
½ tsp ground ginger	0.6	0.08
Sprinkle of nutmeg	—	—
Salt and black pepper to taste	—	—

Preheat oven to 375°F.

Cut squash in half lengthwise. Scoop out seeds and stringy matter in center. Place flesh side down on oiled nonstick baking sheet. Bake for about 1 hour, or until the skin can be punctured with a fork and flesh is soft. Remove from oven and allow to cool a bit, so it can be handled. Scoop out flesh, measuring 4 cups into the workbowl of a food processor and reserving any extra for another purpose. Add remaining ingredients to workbowl and process until smooth. Taste and adjust seasoning. You can add a little cream for creamy texture if desired. Reheat if necessary before serving.

SPAGHETTI SQUASH

You can use spaghetti squash as you would pasta, so feel free to try it with Mushroom Cream Sauce (page 256), or White Clam Sauce (page 255).

8 servings *Per serving: 5.85 gm* CHO, *0.12 oz* PRO

	CHO (gm)	PRO (gm)
1 medium spaghetti squash, 2–3 lb		
(to yield 6 cups cooked squash)	46.8	6.0
Salt and pepper to taste	—	—
Olive oil or butter to toss	—	—

Boil squash whole in water to cover for about 30 minutes, or cut in half and bake flesh side down at 350°F for about 30 minutes, or until skin is tender. Remove seeds and stringy material in center. Scoop out flesh of squash (it too is stringy, but there is a difference). Toss with salt and pepper and enough olive oil or butter to coat. Serve as is, or toss with grated cheese or the sauce of your choice.

PARMESAN-CRUSTED ZUCCHINI

2 servings   *Per serving: 5.75 gm* CHO, *3.34 oz* PRO

	CHO (gm)	PRO (gm)
2 small zucchini, about 8 inches, cut into ¼-inch slices	7.9	1.43
1 egg, slightly beaten	0.6	6.0
¾ cup freshly grated Parmesan cheese	3.0	32.7
Olive oil to fry, about 1 cup	—	—
Salt and pepper to taste	—	—

If you use zucchini without removing some of the moisture, this recipe can turn out soggy. Reducing moisture content is simple — just liberally salt the slices with a shaker, then place on paper towels for about 15 minutes. Heat oil in skillet. It should be hot, simmering, but not boiling hard. Blot zucchini slices dry, dip in egg, then Parmesan. Fry in hot oil until golden brown. Drain on paper towels and season with salt and pepper.

Sauces, Dips, and Dressings

HOLLANDAISE SAUCE

6 servings   *Per serving: 0.39 gm* CHO, *0.31 oz* PRO

	CHO (gm)	PRO (gm)
3 egg yolks	0.9	9.0
1 Tbsp cold water	—	—
Salt and white pepper to taste	—	—
2 sticks butter, cut into small cubes	0.14	2.0
1 Tbsp lemon juice	1.3	0.1

Heat 1 or 2 inches of water in bottom half of a double boiler.
Bring to a simmer, then reduce heat. In top half of double
boiler, combine egg yolks, 1 tablespoon cold water, and salt
and pepper. Place the pan over the hot water and whisk egg
yolks until they begin to thicken. Do not let the mixture get
too hot or the eggs will cook and sauce will become lumpy.
Whisk in butter a few pieces at a time until it is all incorpo-
rated. Whisk until thick and creamy. Whisk in lemon juice.
Makes 1½ cups.

GORGONZOLA SAUCE

6 servings   *Per serving: 1.1 gm* CHO, *0.25 oz* PRO

	CHO (gm)	PRO (gm)
½ tsp finely chopped shallot	0.1	—
⅛ cup crumbled gorgonzola (about ¾ oz)	0.6	4.5
¾ cup heavy cream	6.0	4.8
Freshly ground black pepper	—	—

Combine shallot, gorgonzola, and cream in a skillet. Heat to a simmer. Reduce by half. Season with pepper. Serve with stuffed tenderloin on page 220 or with other roasted or grilled meats. Makes about ½ cup.

MUSTARD SORREL SAUCE

Mint or scallions could be substituted if you can't find sorrel, but the taste will be different.

4 servings   *Per serving: 1.75 gm* CHO, *0.2 oz* PRO

	CHO (gm)	PRO (gm)
3 Tbsp Dijon mustard	—	—
1 Tbsp horseradish	—	—
⅔ cup heavy cream, whipped	5.3	4.24
2 Tbsp lemon zest	1.2	0.2
2 Tbsp chopped sorrel leaves	0.5	0.2
Salt and black pepper to taste	—	—

In a bowl, whisk together Dijon and horseradish. Fold in whipped cream. Mix in lemon zest and sorrel. Season with salt and pepper. Makes about 1½ cups.

AIOLI

8 servings　　　*Per serving: 0.68 gm CHO, 0.14 oz PRO*

	CHO (gm)	PRO (gm)
4 cloves garlic	3.6	0.8
2 egg yolks	0.6	6.0
About 2 cups olive oil, enough to thicken	—	—
2 Tbsp lemon zest	1.2	0.2
1 tsp vinegar	—	—
2 tsp warm water	—	—
Salt and black pepper to taste	—	—

In workbowl of food processor, mince garlic and combine with egg yolks. Process to beat egg yolks. Very slowly, while processing, add olive oil in a thin stream. When you have added about ½ cup oil, start adding lemon zest and vinegar from time to time, still processing. Add 1 teaspoon warm water. Continue to add oil in a slow stream. The mixture should become thick and smooth. Add remaining teaspoon water. Season with salt and pepper. If mixture does not thicken or blend properly, remove aioli from food processor. Put another egg yolk in the workbowl and turn on the machine. Slowly add aioli mixture to egg yolk while processor is running. This procedure should correct sauce. Serve with fish or roasted vegetables. Makes about 2 cups.

PESTO

6 servings   *Per serving: 3.9 gm* CHO, *1* OZ PRO

	CHO (gm)	PRO (gm)
2 cups packed basil leaves	14.4	11.2
3 cloves garlic	2.7	0.6
½ tsp salt, or to taste	—	—
¼ cup pine nuts, toasted	4.4	4.6
½ cup olive oil or to moisten	—	—
½ cup grated Parmesan cheese	2.0	21.8
Salt and black pepper to taste	—	—

Puree the basil, garlic, salt, and pine nuts in a food processor until blended and the mixture becomes a paste. Add the olive oil and blend until the mixture is smooth or to your liking. Add ⅓ cup of the cheese to the mixture, just before serving. The pesto can be frozen before the cheese is added. Reserve the remaining cheese to sprinkle on top when serving. Use pesto with chicken, salmon, or on spaghetti squash. Other herbs can be added — parsley, mint, sorrel, etc. — for a different taste. Makes about 1½ cups.

WHITE CLAM SAUCE

This is good tossed with cooked spaghetti squash (see recipe on page 248).

6 servings   *Per serving: 3 gm* CHO, *2.1 oz* PRO

	CHO (gm)	PRO (gm)
¼ cup olive oil	—	—
¼ cup butter	—	—
2 cloves garlic, minced	1.8	0.2
½ cup water	—	—
½ cup chopped parsley	2.0	0.8
1 tsp salt	—	—
¼ tsp black pepper	—	—
½ tsp dried oregano	0.32	—
16 oz clams, frozen, canned, or fresh, shelled	11.6	58.0
2 Tbsp heavy cream	1.0	0.8
6 Tbsp grated Parmesan cheese (optional)	1.5	16.35

Heat oil and butter in skillet. Sauté garlic over medium heat until lightly browned. Reduce heat. Add water slowly. Reserve 2 Tbsp parsley. Stir in remaining parsley, salt, pepper, and oregano. Add clams and their liquid. Simmer until slightly reduced, about 5 minutes. Stir in cream. Cook a few more minutes, until slightly thickened. Toss with spaghetti squash. Top individual servings with Parmesan and reserved parsley.

MUSHROOM CREAM SAUCE

If you are serving this with spaghetti squash, use the recipe variation on the next page.

4 servings   *Per serving: 4.8 gm* CHO, *0.6 oz* PRO

	CHO (gm)	PRO (gm)
3 Tbsp butter	—	—
¾ lb mushrooms, chopped	14.25	10.59
2 Tbsp chopped shallots	1.8	0.6
6 Tbsp heavy cream	3.0	2.4
Salt and black pepper to taste	—	—

Heat butter in skillet. Sauté mushrooms and shallots until mushrooms begin to brown, about 15 minutes. Add heavy cream. Bring to a simmer. Allow to simmer until the sauce reduces and thickens, 5–10 minutes. Season with salt and pepper. Serve over spaghetti squash into which you have mixed additional butter, cream, and Parmesan (see variation on the next page) or serve with broiled chicken breast. Makes about 2 cups.

Spaghetti Squash Variation

8 servings   Per serving: 8.85 gm CHO, *0.91 gm* PRO

	CHO (gm)	PRO (gm)
2 Tbsp butter	—	—
6 Tbsp heavy cream	3.0	2.4
½ cup grated Parmesan cheese	2.0	21.8
1 recipe Spaghetti Squash (page 248)	46.8	6.0
1 recipe Mushroon Cream Sauce (page 256)	19.05	13.69

Stir butter, cream, and Parmesan into 6 cups hot spaghetti squash. Top with sauce.

ITALIAN-STYLE RED SAUCE*

This sauce can be used in many recipes that call for a red sauce, such as meatloaf or stuffed cabbage. It will keep in the refrigerator 4–5 days. It may be stored in the freezer 2–3 months.

6 servings   *Per serving: 5.6 gm* CHO, *0.36 oz* PRO

	CHO (gm)	PRO (gm)
3 cups diced red bell peppers	27.6	3.6
1 Tbsp olive oil	—	—
¼ cup chopped fresh basil	0.46	0.26
2 cloves garlic, minced	1.8	0.4
1 cup College Inn chicken broth	—	1.0
⅓ cup heavy cream	2.7	2.1
½ tsp salt	—	—
⅓ tsp black pepper	—	—
½ tsp dried oregano	0.3	—
½ tsp stevia powder (1 packet)	—	—
2 Tbsp grated Parmesan cheese	0.5	5.5

In a saucepan, bring a quart of water to a boil. Add diced peppers, cover, and simmer for 20 minutes. Drain liquid from peppers by pouring through a colander. Add peppers to food processor workbowl and puree 2–3 minutes. The finished texture of the puree will contain some pulp. Heat olive oil in a saucepan over a low flame. Add basil and garlic. Sauté

---

*Recipe created by Karen A. Weinstock for *Dr. Bernstein's Diabetes Solution,* 2003 edition.

on a low flame until the aroma is released, 3–4 minutes. Stir in the pepper puree, chicken broth, and heavy cream. While stirring, add remaining seasonings except for grated cheese. Simmer the sauce uncovered for 40 minutes. Add grated cheese to sauce just before serving.

Makes about 3 cups of sauce.

GRILLED ONION GUACAMOLE

6 servings   *Per serving: 2.65 gm* CHO, *0.25 oz* PRO

	CHO (gm)	PRO (gm)
2 slices yellow onion	2.8	0.26
1–2 tsp olive oil	—	—
2 cloves garlic, minced	1.8	0.4
½ small yellow tomato, chopped	0.8	0.35
¼ chili pepper, minced	0.9	0.25
2 small avocados, chopped	7.0	7.4
2 Tbsp fresh lemon juice	2.6	0.2
2 tsp chopped cilantro	—	—
Salt and black pepper to taste	—	—

Brush onion slices with olive oil. Grill or broil until soft and brown on both sides, about 10 minutes. Chop and place in small mixing bowl. Add remaining ingredients and mash together. If the avocado is not quite ripe and the mixture seems a little dry, you can add a little olive oil to give the guacamole a smoother texture. The process can be done in a food processor if you prefer the guacamole smooth instead of chunky. Makes about 2 cups.

PARMESAN DIP

10 servings   *Per serving: 4 gm* CHO, *0.7 oz* PRO

	CHO (gm)	PRO (gm)
1 cup sour cream	9.8	7.3
1 cup mayonnaise	14.4	—
½ green bell pepper, chopped	4.6	0.6
½ cup chopped scallions	4.0	1.0
20 green olives, sliced thin	2.6	0.7
1 Tbsp chopped parsley	0.24	0.11
1 Tbsp chopped basil	0.23	0.13
1 Tbsp fresh oregano leaves	0.6	0.1
½ tsp garlic salt	—	—
¾ cup grated Parmesan cheese	3.0	32.7
Salt and black pepper to taste	—	—

Combine all ingredients. I like this dip chunky. If you want it smoother, you can blend it in a food processor. Refrigerate for several hours. Serve with raw vegetables. Makes about 3½ cups.

BLUE CHEESE DRESSING

20 servings, 4 Tbsp each   Per serving: 2.7 gm CHO, *0.48 oz* PRO

	CHO (gm)	PRO (gm)
½ lb blue cheese	5.6	48.0
1 cup chopped scallions	8.0	2.0
½ cup chopped parsley	2.0	0.8
2 cups mayonnaise	28.8	—
1 cup sour cream	9.8	7.3
½ cup red wine vinegar or cider vinegar	—	—
Salt and black pepper to taste	—	—

Crumble blue cheese. Mix with scallions and parsley. Stir in mayonnaise, sour cream, and vinegar. Season with salt and pepper. Refrigerate overnight. Makes about 5¼ cups.

HORSERADISH DILL MAYONNAISE

8 servings, 2 Tbsp each   *Per serving: 1.8 gm* CHO, *0 gm* PRO

	CHO (gm)	PRO (gm)
1 cup mayonnaise	14.4	—
1½ Tbsp horseradish	—	—
1½ tsp Dijon mustard	—	—
2 drops Tabasco sauce	—	—
2 tsp chopped fresh dill	—	—

Mix all ingredients together with a spoon until well blended. Makes about 1 cup.

DIJON VINAIGRETTE

8 servings, 2 Tbsp each   *Per serving: 0.2 gm* CHO, *0 oz* PRO

	CHO (gm)	PRO (gm)
1 clove garlic, minced	0.9	0.2
1 shallot, minced	0.8	0.3
1 Tbsp Dijon mustard	—	—
1 Tbsp red wine vinegar	—	—
1 cup olive oil	—	—
Salt and black pepper to taste	—	—

Mix together garlic and shallot. Whisk in Dijon and vinegar. Whisk in oil or shake in glass jar with a tight lid. Season generously with salt and pepper. Makes about 1 cup.

CREAMY DRESSING

4 servings, 1½ Tbsp each　　*Per serving: 0.9 gm* CHO, *0 oz* PRO

	CHO (gm)	PRO (gm)
¼ cup mayonnaise	3.6	—
2 tsp flaxseed oil	—	—
2 tsp Dijon mustard	—	—
2 tsp horseradish	—	—
1 tsp chopped parsley	—	—
1 tsp chopped basil (optional)	—	—
Salt and black pepper to taste	—	—

Blend all ingredients together in a bowl, seasoning to taste with salt and pepper. Makes scant ½ cup.

HAZELNUT POPPY SEED DRESSING

12 servings, 2 Tbsp each   Per serving: 0.9 gm CHO, *0.1 oz* PRO

	CHO (gm)	PRO (gm)
¼ cup minced shallots	3.2	1.2
¼ cup red wine vinegar	—	—
1 cup olive oil	—	—
¼ cup poppy seeds	8.0	6.0
2 Tbsp Da Vinci hazelnut syrup, or to taste	—	—
Salt and black pepper to taste	—	—

Combine all ingredients except salt and pepper using a food processor. Season to taste. Makes about 1½ cups.

CRANBERRY RELISH

6 servings   *Per serving: 6.3 gm* CHO, *0.26* OZ PRO

	CHO (gm)	PRO (gm)
1½ cups raw cranberries	20.13	0.6
¾ cup chopped fennel	3.6	1.1
¾ cup pecans, toasted	12.0	7.5
1 Tbsp Da Vinci sugar-free orange syrup, or to taste	—	—
½ tsp cinnamon	0.9	—
Salt and black pepper to taste	—	—
1 Tbsp orange zest	1.3	0.1

For a crunchier relish, chop cranberries, fennel, and pecans together coarsely. Stir in syrup and cinnamon. Add a little salt and pepper to taste. Add orange zest.

For a softer relish, put 2 Tbsp water in small skillet. Add cranberries and fennel. Sauté until just soft. Chop pecans and add, then stir in remaining ingredients. I like this version better than the raw one.

Desserts

PUMPKIN PIE

6 servings   *Per serving: 9 gm* CHO, *0.9 oz* PRO

	CHO (gm)	PRO (gm)
1 cup pecan pieces	15.11	10.0
3 Tbsp melted butter	—	—
1 cup canned pumpkin	19.8	2.7
1 egg	0.6	6.0
6 packets (1 gram each) or tablets stevia, or to taste (see page 156)	—	—
1 tsp cinnamon	1.8	0.1
¼ tsp ground ginger	0.3	—
1 cup heavy cream for filling	8.0	6.4
1 tsp vanilla	0.5	—
1 cup heavy cream for topping	8.0	6.4

Preheat oven to 350°F.

Chop pecans fine in food processor. Add melted butter. Press in bottom of 6-inch pie pan. Bake about 10 minutes.

Combine egg, pumpkin, 5 packets stevia, spices, 1 cup cream, and ½ teaspoon of the vanilla. Mix well. Pour into pecan crust. Bake at 350°F for 30–40 minutes, until set in center. Cool.

Whip 1 cup cream to which 1 packet stevia and ½ teaspoon vanilla have been added. Serve pie topped with whipped cream.

PEANUT BUTTER PIE

8 servings   *Per serving: 3.42 gm* CHO, *0.8 oz* PRO

	CHO (gm)	PRO (gm)
¾ cup pecan pieces	11.33	7.5
2 Tbsp butter, melted	—	—
4 oz cream cheese, softened	4.0	8.0
2½ Tbsp peanut butter	7.5	10.0
1 tsp vanilla	0.5	—
Sweetener to taste: stevia, saccharin, or Equal tablets	—	—
½ cup heavy cream, whipped	4.0	3.2

Grind nuts in grinder or food processor. Mix with butter. Press into 7-inch pie pan.

Mix cream cheese, peanut butter, vanilla, and sweetener in mixer or food processor until well blended. Fold in whipped cream. Transfer mixture into crust. Refrigerate for several hours. The servings are small, but the pie is rich.

SWEET RICOTTA TORTE

6 servings   *Per serving: 4.7 gm* CHO, *2.4 oz* PRO

	CHO (gm)	PRO (gm)
15 oz whole-milk ricotta cheese	14.0	49.0
⅓ cup ground toasted almonds	6.2	6.73
4 eggs	2.4	24.0
1½ Tbsp Da Vinci sugar-free almond syrup	—	—
1½ Tbsp Da Vinci sugar-free vanilla syrup	—	—
1 packet (½ tsp) stevia, or to taste	—	—
2 Tbsp grated coconut	1.5	0.5
⅓ cup heavy cream	2.7	2.13
2 Tbsp sliced and blanched almonds, toasted	1.3	4.0
Butter to grease 9-inch pie pan	—	—

Preheat oven to 350°F.

Mix ricotta and ground almonds. Add eggs, one at a time, mixing each one. Add flavorings, stevia, coconut, and cream. Pour mixture into a buttered 9-inch pie pan. Top with toasted almonds. Bake at 350°F for about 30 minutes.

GINGER CINNAMON CUSTARD

4 servings   *Per serving: 4.6 gm* CHO, *1 oz* PRO

	CHO (gm)	PRO (gm)
2 eggs	1.2	12.0
2 cups heavy cream	16.0	12.4
3 Tbsp Da Vinci sugar-free gingerbread syrup	—	—
½ tsp vanilla	0.25	—
½ tsp cinnamon	0.92	—
Dash salt	—	—

Preheat oven to 350°F.

Beat eggs with hand mixer. Mix in cream. Mix in remaining ingredients. Pour into four 4-ounce custard cups. Bake in water bath (ovenproof pan or dish with about 1 inch of boiling water in it) for about 30 minutes, or until firm in center.

CHOCOLATE MOUSSE

8 servings   *Per serving: 7.9 gm* CHO, *1* OZ PRO

	CHO (gm)	PRO (gm)
4 egg yolks	1.2	12.0
1 Tbsp cognac	—	—
1 Tbsp strong coffee	—	—
6 oz unsweetened chocolate, squares or squeeze packets	51.9	22.4
8 Tbsp (1 stick) soft butter, cut into ½-inch pieces	—	1.0
3 Tbsp Da Vinci sugar-free chocolate syrup	—	—
4 Tbsp Da Vinci sugar-free French vanilla syrup	—	—
2 Tbsp Da Vinci sugar-free orange syrup, or to taste	—	—
4 egg whites	1.2	12.0
¾ cup heavy cream	6.0	4.8
2 Tbsp grated orange zest	2.6	0.2

In a heatproof mixing bowl, beat the egg yolks about 3 minutes, or until they are pale yellow and thick enough to form a ribbon. Beat in the cognac. Set the mixing bowl over a pan of barely simmering water and beat for about 3 minutes, until the eggs are foamy and warm. Then set the bowl over a pan of ice and beat for 3 or 4 minutes or until the mixture is cool again and thick and creamy as mayonnaise.

In the top of a double boiler over simmering water, add the coffee and melt chocolate in it, stirring constantly. When the chocolate has melted completely, beat in the butter, one piece at a time. Add all sweeteners except 1 tablespoon of the vanilla syrup. Beat to form a smooth cream. Beat the chocolate mixture into the egg yolk mixture. Taste for sweetness. In a separate bowl with clean beaters, beat the egg whites until they are stiff enough to form stiff peaks. Stir one-quarter of egg whites into chocolate mixture to lighten it.

Carefully fold in remaining egg whites. Spoon into 8 dessert dishes. Refrigerate for at least 4 hours. Whip cream with remaining tablespoon of vanilla syrup. Top each serving with whipped cream and sprinkle with grated orange zest.

PEANUT BUTTER COOKIES

7 servings   *Per serving: 7.67 gm* CHO, *1.7 oz* PRO

	CHO (gm)	PRO (gm)
2 eggs	1.2	12.0
1 cup natural peanut butter	49.0	56.0
4 Tbsp Da Vinci sugar-free vanilla syrup	—	—
1 tsp vanilla	0.5	—
21 toasted peanut halves	3.0	4.0

Preheat oven to 350°F.

Beat eggs. Add peanut butter. Stir mixture well. Add syrup and vanilla. Put 1-tablespoon mounds of cookie dough on a greased baking sheet in rows, 2 inches apart. Top each cookie with a peanut half. Bake 10 minutes. Makes 21 cookies.

Fudge Variation

Substitute Da Vinci sugar-free chocolate syrup for vanilla syrup to make Peanut Butter Fudge Cookies.

WALNUT SWEETMEATS

6 servings   *Per serving: 2.06 gm CHO, 0.48 oz PRO*

	CHO (gm)	PRO (gm)
1 cup walnut halves	13.7	15.2
2 Tbsp Da Vinci sugar-free hazelnut or French vanilla syrup	—	—
2 Tbsp melted butter (optional)	—	—
¼ tsp cinnamon, or to taste	0.45	—
Salt to taste	—	—

Preheat oven to 350°F.

Toss walnuts with syrup and optional butter until well coated. Sprinkle with cinnamon and salt. Bake at 350°F about 10 minutes, or until they look toasted. Eat plain or add to salads in lieu of croutons or for an added crunch.

Pecan Variation

6 servings   *Per serving: 2.3 gm CHO, 0.25 oz PRO*

Substitute 1 cup pecan halves (13.72 gm CHO, 9.08 gm PRO) for the walnuts, and use Da Vinci sugar-free caramel syrup instead of hazelnut or French vanilla.

VANILLA CREAM SODA

1 serving   *Per serving: 1 gm* CHO, *0.13 oz* PRO

	CHO (gm)	PRO (gm)
Club soda to fill glass	—	—
2 Tbsp Da Vinci sugar-free vanilla syrup	—	—
2 Tbsp heavy cream	1.0	0.8

Fill large glass with ice. Add club soda, leaving room for syrup and cream. Add syrup. Stir to blend. Add cream.

Recipe Index

General Index

About the Author

Richard K. Bernstein, M.D., is recognized as one of the foremost experts on diabetes and its complications. His private practice in Mamaroneck, New York, is devoted solely to diabetes and prediabetic conditions such as obesity. He is a Fellow of the American College of Nutrition and of the American College of Endocrinology and is a Diplomate of the American Academy of Wound Management. He is director of the Peripheral Vascular Disease Clinic of the Albert Einstein College of Medicine and is a member of the American Medical Writers Association and the National Association of Science Writers. He has written five books on diabetes and many articles in scientific and popular journals.

The Web site for Dr. Bernstein's current books is www.diabetes-book.com.